THE

ULTIMATE

POCKET

DIET

JOURNAL

WORKS WITH ALL DIET PROGRAMS!

BY ALEX LLUCH

THE ULTIMATE POCKET DIET JOURNAL
By Alex Lluch

Copyright © 2006
By Wedding Solutions Publishing, Inc.
San Diego, California 92119

ALL RIGHTS RESERVED

All rights reserved under International and Pan-American Copyright Conventions. No part of this publication may be reproduced, stored in a retrieval system, or transmitted in any form or by any means, electronic or mechanical, including photocopying, recording or by any information storage and retrieval system without prior permission from Wedding Solutions Publishing, Inc.

Nutritional and fitness guidelines based on information provided by the United States Food and Drug Administration, Food and Nutrition Information Center, National Agricultural Library, Agricultural Research Service, and the U.S. Department of Agriculture.

Cover Image: Photodisc Red Collection/Getty Images

ISBN-13: 978-1-887169-56-1
Printed in China

DISCLAIMER: The content in this book is provided for general informational purposes only and is not meant to substitute for the advice provided by a medical professional. This information is not intended to diagnose or treat medical problems or substitute for appropriate medical care. If you are under the care of a physician and/or take medications for diabetes, heart disease, hypertension, or any other medications, consult your health care provider prior to initiation of any dietary program. Implementation of a dietary program may require altercation in your medication needs and must be done by or under the direction of your physician. If you have or suspect that you have a medical problem, promptly contact your health care provider. Never disregard professional medical advice or delay in seeking it because of something you have read in this book.

Wedding Solutions Publishing, Inc. makes no claims whatsoever regarding the interpretation or utilization of any information contained herein and/or recorded by the user of this journal. If you utilize any information provided in this book, you do so at your own risk and you specifically waive any right to make any claim against the author and publisher, its officers, directors, employees or representatives as the result of the use of such information. Consult your physician before making any changes in your diet or exercise.

TABLE OF CONTENTS

TABLE OF CONTENTS

INTRODUCTION

By purchasing this book, you have taken the first step in your weight-loss journey to looking and feeling great. Whether you are a veteran of the diet game, or in search of a comprehensive weight-loss program, this is the right book for you!

More than half of American adults today are overweight, with one-third considered obese. America's weight problem has become a serious issue because of the increasing number of diseases linked to being overweight, such as high cholesterol, high blood pressure, diabetes, stroke, and heart disease. Such diseases can reduce the quality of life and, in some cases, lead to death. In America, obesity causes roughly 300,000 deaths each year, while healthcare costs of adults who are obese continue to rise. Several factors can contribute to being overweight, including family genetics, the growing portion sizes of food, and the tendency to overeat. The most common way to determine whether or not a person is obese is through Body Mass Index, or BMI. This is a ratio of a person's height and weight, and when a person's BMI is over 25, he or she can be considered overweight. Unfortunately, BMIs over 25 are an increasing trend in America's health statistics. We are a nation whose waistline is expanding, and will continue to grow unless we take control of our eating and exercise habits.

Losing weight has major benefits that can improve your way of life. Weight-loss can lower the risk of the diseases mentioned above, help you become healthy and more active, and also make you look and feel better about yourself. It is difficult in today's society to make the right choices regarding your health and diet. Food portions in restaurants are larger, which encourage us to eat more; our jobs promote sedentary lifestyles; and fast food, while often unhealthy, is convenient and inexpensive. Many food companies use larger sized portions as selling points, making the claim that bigger is better. It then becomes the consumer's responsibility to monitor how much he or she eats and to know how much is personally enough. That is where this journal comes in: it educates you on proper weight management and weight-loss methods. It provides important dietary and health information, and it helps you make the right decisions to begin your weight-loss plan so you can uncover a healthier, better-looking you!

By using this diet journal, you are taking charge of your weight-loss program. It is a useful resource of nutritional information and fitness guidelines and will help you assess your current weight and health status. Another advantage of this book is that it will guide you in setting down an appropriate plan for yourself. It also makes counting calories and keeping track of nutritional values simple.

Being aware of what you eat is an important step in the direction of weight-loss: it keeps you responsible for everything you consume, creating an on-going awareness of your diet program. When you write down everything you eat, you hold yourself accountable for your food consumption, so not even the tiniest bite of a cookie should slip by!

In addition, this journal will help you keep track of your daily progress as you move closer towards your weight-loss goal. This on-going routine will make your program more effective. With this journal as your companion, you can make better, more informed choices that will help you lose weight, look better, and improve your health!

Congratulations!

HOW TO USE THIS
DIET JOURNAL

Each section of this diet journal is specifically designed to help guide you through the various stages of your weight-loss program. It will allow you to assess your current health, identify eating behaviors and patterns that may prevent you from losing weight, provide proper nutrition and fitness guidelines, and help you create realistic goals and expectations as you go through your journey to look better and improve your health.

ASSESSING YOUR WEIGHT & HEALTH STATUS

Before you begin your quest, it is imperative to define your starting point, as well as your final goal. You can calculate your current status in height, weight, and Body Mass Index (BMI), and assess your health risks based on your genetic predisposition and family history. You should also investigate behaviors that may have led to your current weight situation, such as emotional triggers, guilt-based eating, and stress snacking.

DEVELOPING A SUCCESSFUL
WEIGHT-LOSS PROGRAM

When developing your personal weight-loss program, you should keep in mind five main concepts: Motivation, Realistic Timelines, Personal Success, Visualization, and Maintenance. Reflecting on these essential points will help you determine the program that is individualized for your needs. Once you have defined these terms in relation to your own goals, you can establish additional habits that will assist you on your weight-loss journey.

Writing in your diet journal should become part of your daily routine. Be sure to take full advantage of your program by documenting the foods and beverages you consume in your journal. This way you will be able to stay motivated and keep track of your daily calorie allowance, nutritional value intake, and weight-loss progress.

THINGS YOU SHOULD KNOW TO LOSE WEIGHT

Nutritional Guidelines: Start your program armed with information on the USDA Food Guide and the Nutrition Facts label. This book will help you become an expert on food facts. Included in this journal are nutritional values for over 1,000 popular food items. This information will help you break down the nutritional content of the foods you eat during your diet. You will learn how to count calories and determine how sugar, sodium, cholesterol, carbohydrates, fats, and protein affect your body. By using this book, you will shed those unwanted pounds and be on your way to improved health.

Physical Activity: Burning calories through physical activity is a great way to expedite a successful weight-loss program. Physical activities can transform your body to a higher level of fitness and help you feel great.

YOUR PERSONAL PROFILE

Fill out your personal health profile at the start of your diet so you can accurately assess your current physical state, habits, and eating patterns. Documenting this information will assist you in identifying the areas of your diet and health that need improvement. If in doubt, consult with a professional so you can receive medical clearance to begin a safe diet and fitness program.

YOUR PERSONAL WEIGHT-LOSS GOALS, PLANS & ACHIEVEMENTS

In this section, you will solidify your weight-loss goals and plans. You will be able to write down the specific targets you want to reach and the means you will take to achieve them. Be sure to establish realistic weight-loss goals that are broken down into daily, weekly, and monthly objectives.

You will also be able to document your results at the end of your program. Keep in mind that consistent effort and steady progress will help you achieve your target weight. You will be amazed at your weight-loss progress, reduced body-fat percentage, and new measurements. Take "before" and "after" photos to visually document your successful efforts.

THE SECRET TO WEIGHT-LOSS:
KEEPING TRACK OF WHAT YOU EAT

This section is the heart of your program because it is crucial to your weight-loss success. It is a source of personal feedback and a comprehensive daily reminder of all of the elements of your weight-loss plan. Your daily journal can help you stay focused on your personal goals and keep you motivated towards your weight-loss target. These pages will help you keep track of your food and beverage intake, make sure you are within your daily calorie allotment, and ensure that you are getting enough fluids. You will also be able to log your physical fitness activities, supplements, energy levels, and daily weight.

OTHER GREAT FEATURES OF
THIS DIET JOURNAL

YOUR WEIGHT-LOSS PROGRESS CHART

Chart your daily, weekly, and/or monthly progress as you gradually achieve your weight-loss goals. This is an exciting way to map your progress towards a new and healthier you.

Customize the chart according to your personal weight-loss goals. Begin by recording your current weight in the far left column where it states "Start Here/Enter Weight." This marker provides enough space above and below your current weight to allow for fluctuation.

The horizontal lines of the graph signify pounds of weight. Decide how many pounds each horizontal line should indicate. For example, if you have alot of weight to lose, you will probably want each horizontal line to indicate one pound. So if your starting weight is 170, you would write this down next to "Start Here/Enter Weight." If you want to lose 20 pounds, you would use each line to mark one pound of weight. Proceed to fill in the rest of the numbers on the left column. The line directly under your current weight would be 169 and would decrease until you reach your goal weight of 150. The lines above your current weight would start with 171 and up, to allow for fluctuation.

For moderate weight-loss, use every other line to record each pound. If you only have a minimal amount of weight to lose, you can use the dark-blue horizontal lines to indicate one pound.

The vertical lines indicate days of the week. You have the option of plotting your progress on a daily, weekly, or monthly basis. Each dark blue vertical line indicates the first day of each week. To chart your progress, simply locate the vertical line at the bottom of the page that corresponds to the day of your program. Follow the line until you reach your weight for the day on the left column. Mark that point. Repeat for each day or week of your program. As you progress through your program, connect the points to create a visual graph of your weight-loss.

NUTRITIONAL FACTS ON POPULAR FOOD ITEMS

This section is a great resource of nutritional information on foods you may want to select for your weight-loss program. It provides calories per serving as well as nutritional content for fat, protein, carbohydrates, and fiber.

To use this section, look up food items listed in alphabetical order. Locate the corresponding information, and log the data into your journal so you can keep track of your daily totals.

ASSESSING YOUR WEIGHT
& HEALTH STATUS

The most important reasons to start a weight-loss program are to look and feel great, as well as reduce the risk of health complications, such as heart disease and diabetes. Before you start, however, it is important to assess your health status. There are three methods to determine your overall physical condition: your height and weight measurements, waist size, and Body Mass Index (BMI). Another consideration is your family history.

For adults 18 years and older, the first step is to measure your height and weight. Use those two numbers to find your BMI on the following page. If your BMI falls within the range of 19 to 24, you are considered healthy. If your BMI lands from 24 to 29, then you are at increased risk of developing health problems. If your BMI is 30 or above, you could be considered obese. If you fall into the last two categories, it is essential to plan and manage your weight-loss program.

The second factor in evaluating your weight is your waist size. Use a tape measure to calculate your waist circumference below your rib cage and above your belly button. You have an increased health risk for developing serious chronic illness if your waist size is more than 35 inches for women and 40 inches for men. For more information, see the chart on page 17.

Your personal history and family background can shed additional light on possible health risks. Be aware of increased potential problems if your family history includes arthritis, high blood pressure, high cholesterol, high blood sugar, death at a young age, heart problems, cancer, or respiratory illness. A history of family illness doesn't mean these conditions are destined to be a part of your future, but is yet another reason to get started on the road to good health and physical fitness.

BODY MASS INDEX - BMI

Body composition can vary greatly from individual to individual. Two people who possess the same height and weight can have different bone structure and varying percentages of muscle and fat. Therefore, your weight alone is not the only factor in assessing your risk for weight related health issues. Your BMI can help indicate whether or not your health is at risk.

Calculating your BMI: Locate your height in the left hand column on the following page. Then move across the row to your weight. The number at the very top of the column is your BMI.

BMI	19	20	21	22	23	24	25	26	27	28	29	30	31	32	33	34	35
Height								weight in pounds									
4'10"	91	96	100	105	110	115	119	124	129	134	138	143	148	153	158	162	167
4'11"	94	99	104	109	114	119	124	128	133	138	143	148	153	158	163	168	173
5'	97	102	107	112	118	123	128	133	138	143	148	153	158	163	158	174	179
5'1"	100	106	111	116	122	127	132	137	143	148	153	158	164	169	174	180	185
5'2"	104	109	115	120	126	131	136	142	147	153	158	164	169	175	180	186	191
5'3"	107	113	118	124	130	135	141	146	152	158	163	169	175	180	186	191	197
5'4"	110	116	122	128	134	140	145	151	157	163	169	174	180	186	192	197	204
5'5"	114	120	126	132	138	144	150	156	162	168	174	180	186	192	198	204	210
5'6"	118	124	130	136	142	148	155	161	167	173	179	186	192	198	204	210	216
5'7"	121	127	134	140	146	153	159	166	172	178	185	191	198	204	211	217	223
5'8"	125	131	138	144	151	158	164	171	177	184	190	197	203	210	216	223	230
5'9"	128	135	142	149	155	162	169	176	182	189	196	203	209	216	223	230	236
5'10"	132	139	146	153	160	167	174	181	188	195	202	209	216	222	229	236	243
5'11"	136	143	150	157	165	172	179	186	193	200	208	215	222	229	236	243	250
6'	140	147	154	162	169	177	184	191	199	206	213	221	228	235	242	250	258
6'1"	144	151	159	166	174	182	189	197	204	212	219	227	235	242	250	257	265
6'2"	148	155	163	171	179	186	194	202	210	218	225	233	241	249	256	264	272
6'3"	152	160	168	176	184	192	200	208	216	224	232	240	248	256	264	272	279
	Healthy						Overweight					Obese					

IS YOUR WEIGHT A HEALTH RISK?

For most adults, BMI and waist size are relatively reliable ways to indicate whether or not you are overweight. These two indicators are also effective in assessing your risk of weight related health issues.

Your waist measurement determines whether or not you have the tendency to carry fat around your midsection. A higher waist size may indicate a greater risk for weight related health issues such as high blood pressure, Type 2 diabetes and coronary artery disease. Typically, the higher your Body Mass Index, the greater risk to your health. This risk also increases if your waist is greater than 35 inches for women or 40 inches for men.

If your weight indicates that you are at a higher risk for health problems, consult your primary care physician to determine safe and effective ways to improve your health. Even moderate amounts of weight-loss, around 5-10 percent of your weight, can have long lasting health benefits as long as you keep off the pounds.

Risk of Associated Disease According to BMI and Waist Size

Body Mass Index		Waist less than or equal to 40" Men 35" Women	Waist greater than 40" Men 35" Women
18 or less	Underweight	N/A	N/A
19-24	Normal	N/A	N/A
25-29	Overweight	Increased	High
30-35	Obese	High	Very High
over 35	Obese	Very High	Very High

IDENTIFY YOUR EATING PATTERNS

Changing your eating habits requires adjusting your attitude toward food. Begin by understanding the situations and emotional triggers that lead to overeating. Let's take a look at some common behaviors:

Are you compelled to eat as an emotional response to your thoughts and feelings? If you eat when you're upset, frustrated, angry, lonely, or tired, the answer most likely is yes. Food feels like the perfect temporary solution – that is, until it is finished, and then guilt sets in because the food choice may not have been healthy. Try to choose other behaviors as an emotional response, such as taking a walk or calling a friend.

Do you eat when you are not hungry because you think you should? Sometimes the time of day is enough encouragement to eat a meal or a quick snack, despite a lack of actual physical hunger. Instead, learn to listen to your body. If you are not hungry, you shouldn't eat.

Do you feel guilty leaving food on your plate? Perhaps when you were a child, you were told to finish all of the food on your plate. This sense of guilt should no longer gauge how much food you should eat. It is acceptable to stop eating when you feel full.

Do you make poor food choices because of peer pressure? It is far easier to go with the flow when those around you are eating unhealthy foods. It takes self-control and determination to follow your weight-loss plan at social gatherings or all-you-can-eat buffets. Congratulate yourself when you stick to your plan and successfully fend off unhealthy snacking urges.

Do you eat out of boredom? Food can become a time-filler when you are bored. Don't fall into this trap! Try to motivate yourself and choose a fun and interesting activity as an alternative to snacking. If you are otherwise occupied with an activity where food is not involved, it will be easier to wait for your regularly scheduled meal.

DEVELOPING A SUCCESSFUL

WEIGHT-LOSS PROGRAM

PERSONAL SUCCESS

Reaching your personal goals for your weight-loss program starts with the desire for success. As you move through each phase of your plan, the definition of success can take on many different meanings. In the previous sections, success could be found in honestly assessing your weight and health status. Now is the time to fine-tune your personal interpretation of success by defining how the following key points can help you achieve your weight-loss goal.

Motivation: Your journey takes on a new challenge as you look at the reasons behind your desire for personal success. The first component is to discover your source of motivation. What are your top three reasons for pursuing your weight-loss goal? Write them down in this journal and read them often as a reminder and a source of inspiration. They will help you stay focused on your future weight-loss goals.

Realistic Timelines: The second component is to set realistic goals for yourself. Select a healthy plan and allow an appropriate length of time for your program to succeed. Promises of quick weight-loss may sound too good to be true and most likely are unhealthy and possibly dangerous. General guidelines for healthy weight-loss suggest losing 1 to 2 pounds per week.

Personal Success: The third component is to focus on the positive aspects of your weight-loss. Try to celebrate small achievements along the way so you can stay motivated towards your long term goal. These personal achievements will help you keep a positive attitude. By writing these successes in your daily journal, you can acknowledge your accomplishments whether they are baby steps or huge leaps of progress.

Visualization: A mental picture is worth a thousand words. In your mind's eye, envision your weight-loss before it happens. Visualize all aspects of the new you from your appearance to your improved health. Remember, if you can see it, chances are very good you can make that healthy visual a reality.

Maintenance: The fifth and final component is maintaining your weight-loss long after you have achieved your goal. Remember to stick with the healthy behaviors, habits, and attitudes that led you to your goal. Keep up the good work, for there is nothing more gratifying than maintaining an ideal weight and a healthy lifestyle!

WRITING FOR WEIGHT-LOSS SUCCESS

Writing in your daily diet journal should be a key factor for your weight-loss program. It will help you stick to your routine, stay focused, and realize your personal goals. This journal will make it easy to keep track of your food and beverage intake, water consumption, and physical activities.

Weight: Your daily weight is an excellent source of feedback. If you do not own a scale, this is the perfect time to buy one. Each morning before eating breakfast, step on the scale and write that number in your daily journal. This is one of the ways you will be able to track your success during your weight-loss program. Try not to be discouraged if your progress is slow or the scale indicates a weight gain. It is normal for your body to fluctuate within a 1-to-2 pound range possibly due to water retention. Stick with your weight-loss plans because you will see success over the course of weeks and months.

Count Your Calories: Each morning, afternoon, and evening write down all the foods you eat including added sauces, condiments, and seasonings. Don't forget your snacks and beverages because every calorie counts. Log the portion size and the corresponding calories for that amount of food. Calculate the calories per meal, and at the end of the day, determine the total calories you have consumed. Compare that number to your daily goal. If you were over your target number, don't penalize yourself. Simply try again tomorrow.

This information is vital to your success because it will help you to identify your strengths and weaknesses, discover your eating patterns, and make healthy food selections.

Nutrition Facts: In addition to counting calories, it is important to keep an eye on the nutritional value of your food choices. Read food labels or consult the Nutritional Facts section located in the back of this book to find information on fat, carbohydrates, protein and fiber content. Keep tabs on all of your nutritional totals in your daily journal, as it may indicate future adjustments for food selections.

THINGS YOU SHOULD KNOW
TO LOSE WEIGHT

SUGGESTED DAILY CALORIES FOR WEIGHT MAINTENANCE AND WEIGHT-LOSS

Your total daily calories should be based on your age, gender, body type, and level of physical activity. Here are some suggested daily calorie goals for healthy U.S. adults who are maintaining their ideal weight: active men should consume approximately 2,800 calories per day, active women and sedentary men should eat 2,200 calories, and sedentary women and older adults should strive for 1,600 calories. If you are not sure of how many daily calories you should consume, consult your primary care physician for a recommendation.

The total number of daily calories for a weight-loss plan will depend on the number of pounds you wish to lose. Once you have determined the daily number of calories that you should eat to maintain your weight, you should decrease your total caloric intake by an average of 500 calories per day for a moderate weight-loss. To proceed in a safe and healthy manner, you can eliminate those 500 calories simply by decreasing the amount of sugars, refined carbohydrates, and alcohol in your diet, most of which provide calories with little nutritional value.

RECOMMENDED DAILY AMOUNT FROM EACH FOOD GROUP

The United States Department of Agriculture is known for its Food Guide, which is a nutritional reference for many health groups and dietary plans. The USDA Food Guide separates the foods you should eat into 6 different categories: fruits, vegetables, grains, lean meat and beans, milk, and oils. The suggested amounts below have been developed to help you select the proper amount of food to eat from each group on a daily basis. Each group provides you with a different set of essential nutrients. By following the recommended serving sizes, you can be assured that you are getting the proper amounts of protein, fats, carbohydrates, fiber, vitamins, and minerals. This guide can be adjusted to suit your personal needs.

Calorie Level	1,200	1,400	1,600	1,800	2,000	2,200	2,400	2,600	2,800	3,000
Food Group	Food group amounts shown in cup (C) or ounce (oz), with number of servings (srv) in parentheses. Oils are shown in grams									
Fruits	1 C (2 srv)	1.5 C (3 srv)	1.5 C (3 srv)	1.5 C (3 srv)	2 C (4 srv)	2 C (4 srv)	2 C (4 srv)	2 C (4 srv)	2.5 C (5 srv)	2.5 C (5 srv)
Vegetables	1.5 C (3 srv)	1.5 C (3 srv)	2 C (4 srv)	2.5 C (5 srv)	2.5 C (5 srv)	3 C (6 srv)	3 C (6 srv)	3.5 C (7 srv)	3.5 C (7 srv)	4 C (8 srv)
Grains	4 oz	5 oz	5 oz	6 oz	6 oz	7 oz	8 oz	9 oz	10 oz	10 oz
Lean Meat & Beans	3 oz	4 oz	5 oz	5 oz	5.5 oz	6 oz	6.5 oz	6.5 oz	7 oz	7 oz
Milk	2 C	2 C	3 C	3 C	3 C	3 C	3 C	3 C	3 C	3 C
Oils	17 g	17 g	22 g	24 g	27 g	29 g	31 g	34 g	36 g	44 g

THE NUTRITION FACTS LABEL

Most packaged foods have a nutrition facts label. Use this information to make healthy choices quickly and easily.

LABEL AT A GLANCE

Nutrition Facts

Serving Size 1 cup (228g)
Servings Per Container 2

Amount per Serving

Calories 250   Calories from Fat 110

	% Daily Value*
Total Fat 12g	**18%**
Saturated Fat 3g	**15%**
Trans Fat 3g	
Cholesterol 30mg	**10%**
Sodium 470mg	**20%**
Total Carbohydrate 31g	**10%**
Dietary Fiber 0g	**0%**
Sugars 5g	
Protein 5g	

Vitamin A	**4%**
Vitamin C	**2%**
Calcium	**20%**
Iron	**4%**

* Percent Daily Values are based on a 2,000 calorie diet. Your Daily Values may be higher or lower depending on your calorie needs.

	Calories:	2,000	2,500
Total Fat	Less than	65g	80g
Sat Fat	Less than	20g	25g
Cholesterol	Less than	300mg	300mg
Sodium	Less than	2,400mg	2,400mg
Total Carbohydrate		300g	375g
Dietary Fiber		25g	30g

Start Here: Check the serving size and servings per container

Calories: 400 or more calories per serving is considered high. Note the calories from fat.

Daily Values: 5%=low, 20%=high

Limit These Nutrients: Eating too much fat, saturated fat, trans fat, cholesterol, or sodium may put you at an increased health risk for diseases such as heart disease, some cancers, or high blood pressure.

Get Enough of These Nutrients: Most Americans do not receive the proper amount of fiber, vitamins A, C, calcium or iron from their diets. Eating enough of these nutrients can limit your risk of diseases such as osteoporosis and heart disease.

Daily Values Footnote: This footnote makes recommendations for key nutrients based on diets of 2,000 and 2,500 daily calories.

A BREAKDOWN OF THE NUTRITION FACTS LABEL

The first place to look when selecting foods at the market is the product label. Check out "Nutrition Facts" for the ingredient list, serving size, calories, amounts, nutrients, portions, and percentage of daily nutritional values. Often you will see "enriched" food sources for wheat or pasta. This is an indication that vitamins or minerals have been added for nutrition. Commonly added nutrients are calcium, thiamin, riboflavin, niacin, iron, and folic acid. The ingredient list tells you exactly what is in the food including nutrients and whether fat or sugar have been added. The ingredients are also listed in descending order by weight.

What Is a Serving Size?: When hunger strikes and a type of food calls out to you, it is important to look at the label for serving size information. The Nutrition Facts label indicates the quantity of food per portion and the number of servings in the package. Serving sizes are now standardized to make it easier to compare foods in familiar units like cups, pieces, grams, or metric amounts. According to the sample label on the previous page, one serving of food equals one cup containing 250 calories. If you ate the whole package, you would have consumed two cups or 500 calories.

All Calories Are Not Created Equal: Calories provide a concrete measure of how much energy you receive from a serving size of a selected food. If you are overweight, chances are you consume more calories than your body needs on a daily basis. You should also be aware of how many calories per serving come from fat. In the sample label, there are 250 calories in a serving, and 110 of those come from fat. That means almost half of the calories are from fat. If you ate two servings or 500 calories, 220 would come from fat, which is 44 percent. To lose weight, select foods with 20 percent or less calories from fat per serving. These can be from proteins, dairy products, and whole grain breads, cereals, and pasta. Most fresh fruits and vegetables are naturally low in fat.

Keep Tabs on Cholesterol: Cholesterol is a fat-like substance present in all animal foods, such as meat, poultry, fish, milk and milk products, and egg yolks. It's a good idea to select lean meats, avoid eating the skin of poultry, and use low-fat milk products. Egg yolks and organ meats, like liver, are high in cholesterol. Plant foods, such as fruit and vegetables, do not contain cholesterol. Why is this important information? Eating foods high in dietary cholesterol increases blood cholesterol in many people, which increases their risk for heart disease. Most health authorities suggest dietary cholesterol should be limited to 300 mg or less per day.

Salt and Sodium: It's important to include some salt in your diet, but it should be limited to 2,400 mg per day. You can keep track of your daily intake by looking at the Nutrition Facts label. Go easy on luncheon and cured meats, cheeses, canned soups and vegetables, and soy sauce. Look for no-salt-added products at your supermarket. Be cautious and avoid adding table salt to your food. Each teaspoon of salt adds 2,000 mg of sodium to your diet. So put down the salt shaker and re-train your taste buds.

Sugar - How Sweet it Isn't: Sugar is an ingredient that is found in almost every food product. If you are counting calories, it is important to look at the list of ingredients to identify all sources of sugar. Obvious foods that add sugar are jams, ice cream, canned fruit and chocolate milk. You will also find it in cereals, sauces, frozen foods, and salad dressings. Here's a list of common sweeteners that are essentially sugar: white sugar, honey, sucrose, fructose, maltose, lactose, syrup, corn syrup, high-fructose corn syrup, molasses, and fruit-juice concentrate. If these terms are found in the first four listings on the label, that food is likely to be very high in sugar. Hint: labels are listed in grams. Consider 4 grams to equal 1 teaspoon of sugar. Total daily intake for all added sugar sources not found naturally in the food itself, should be a maximum 6 teaspoons a day.

Carbohydrates: Breads, cereals, rice, and pasta provide carbohydrates, which are excellent sources of energy. If you are on a weight-loss plan, it is important to include them in your diet because they provide vitamins, minerals, and fiber. One serving of carbohydrates equals one slice of bread, one ounce of ready- to-eat cereal, or 1/2 cup cooked cereal, rice or pasta. Focus on complex carbohydrates, such as whole grain breads, cereals, and brown rice. Keep these foods healthy by not adding additional butter, margarine, cream, cheese, sugar, oils, and fat. Limit refined carbohydrates, such as white flour and sugar, as well as processed foods like pre-packaged candy, cookies, cakes, and chips.

Fruits & Vegetables: Fruits and vegetables can be works of art if you select a rainbow of nine colorful choices throughout your day. For example, eat a yellow banana, green broccoli, orange carrots, a red apple, purple cabbage, and blueberries. Rotate your selections to get the most from your foods. Fruits and vegetables provide vitamins A, C, and folate, and minerals like iron, potassium, and magnesium. Keep in mind that it is important to eat these foods as fresh as possible, preferably raw, and avoid adding butter, mayonnaise, and high-fat salad dressings. When possible, choose the actual piece of fruit, like an apple, over juice.

Protein: The USDA Food Guide suggests eating cooked lean meat as a source of protein for optimum health. Protein provides an essential supply of B vitamins, zinc, and iron. Make sure you get enough of these nutrients by combining a variety of choices, such as lean cuts of beef, pork, veal, lamb, chicken, turkey, fish, and shellfish. Other protein possibilities are eggs, beans, nut butters, tofu, dried nuts, and seeds. Try to choose lean cuts of meat, remove the skin from poultry, trim away all visible fat, go easy on egg yolks, and eat nuts and seeds sparingly.

Fat: As a food source, fat supplies energy and essential fatty acids to your body. Fat-soluble vitamins like A, D, E, K and carotenoids need fat to be absorbed into the body. Not all types of fat are healthy, however, especially saturated fats found in whole milk, butter, ice cream, poultry skin, and palm oil. Unsaturated fats, found mainly in vegetable oils, do not increase blood cholesterol.

A third category called Trans Fat is formed when liquid oils are made into solid fats, like shortening and hard margarine. This type of fat is dangerous because it raises blood cholesterol and increases the risk of coronary heart disease, which is one of the leading causes of death in the United States. Foods high in Trans Fat are processed foods made with partially hydrogenated vegetable oils, such as vegetable shortenings. These oils can be found in crackers, cookies, candies, snack foods, fried foods, and baked goods. It is difficult to avoid all foods with Trans Fat so the ideal goal would be to limit your intake of processed foods as much as possible.

Foods With Healthy Sources of Fat: Try choosing vegetable oils like olive, canola, soybean, sunflower, and corn. Avoid coconut and palm kernel oils. Consider adding fish to your menu twice a week. Salmon and mackerel have omega-3 fatty acids, which offer protection against heart disease. Choose lean meats like skinless chicken, lean beef, and pork. Avoid all fried foods. Watch your fat calories because they contain nine calories per gram, compared to carbohydrates and protein, which have only four calories per gram.

A COMPLETE PHYSICAL FITNESS PROGRAM

Your mission is to burn calories. Your new fitness program should include three essential elements for successful, long-term weight-loss and maintenance: the first element is to include aerobic activities, which provide cardiovascular benefits; the second element is a resistance or strength training program for improving muscle tone; and the third element is to consider integrating a basic stretching routine into your daily schedule to develop flexibility.

Before embarking on your mission, see a doctor to obtain a health clearance if you have unique health issues, injuries, or physical limitations. When you are ready to exercise, warm up slowly and be gentle to your body. It's the only one you've got, so take care of it as you work your way into top physical form.

Aerobic Activities: An aerobic activity is any type of body movement that speeds up your heart rate and breathing. It improves your ability to utilize oxygen, which increases your cardiovascular health. You can participate in aerobic activities almost anywhere, step classes at a gym, running in a park or on a stationary bicycle in your home environment. The minimum amount of time for adult daily exercise is 30 minutes, and children benefit from 60 minutes per day. Keep in mind these numbers are a general estimate and should be tailored to fit individual needs. In all cases, use common sense when exercising and be sure to listen to your body. A general guideline for physical activity is to safely challenge your body while gradually stretching your limits.

Resistance & Strength Training: Once you have a personalized aerobic program that fits your style, consider adding a crucial piece of the puzzle to your fitness regime. Resistance and strength training will firm up muscles as the unwanted pounds melt away. This type of exercise should be done for 20 to 30 minutes, three times a week. It includes lifting hand-held weights, using machines at a gym, or working out with videos in your home. If you choose to go to the gym, consult with professionals and learn how to correctly use the equipment.

Stretching & Flexibility: Stretching and flexibility are often neglected components of physical activity. Preparing the body for movement, and keeping it injury-free, should be built into every fitness program. Stretching and flexibility training is designed to develop range of motion, increase muscle elasticity, and achieve muscle balance. Stretching can also speed up recovery in preparation for the next fitness session. You should never stretch your body when it's cold or stiff. Be sure to start your physical activity with 10 to 15 minutes of slow movement until your muscles have warmed up. Mild stretching can be done at a mid-point in your daily training and again at the completion of the exercise program.

The best type of overall stretching routine is one that starts with the head and neck, working down towards the toes. It uses slow stretches that are held for a minimum of 10 seconds each. Avoid quick-pulling motions that put stress on muscles and joints. Choose abdominal exercises that support the lower back region. In all cases, consult with a professional for advice before beginning a strength and flexibility program.

EXERCISE AND WEIGHT CONTROL

Carrying around too much body fat is a nuisance. Many people fight the "battle of the bulge" through diet alone because exercise is not always convenient. Few of today's occupations require physical activity and many people spend hours behind desks and computers. In addition, much of our leisure time is spent in sedentary pursuits. To reverse this trend, it is important to adjust your attitude and find time to exercise each day. Here's a look at the most common reasons people use to avoid physical activity:

1. I don't have the time.
2. I'm too tired and I don't feel like it.
3. I'm not very good at exercising.
4. It's not convenient to get to my workout place.
5. I'm afraid and embarrassed.

Overweight or Overfat?: Being overweight and overfat are two different dilemmas. Some people, such as athletes, have a muscular physique and weigh more than average for their age and height, but their body composition, which is the amount of fat versus lean body mass (muscle, bone, organs and tissue), is within an acceptable range. Others can weigh within the range of U.S. guidelines, yet can carry around too much fat. Use exercise as a way to balance your body fat percentage. An easy self-test is to pinch the thickness of fat at your waist and abdomen. If you can pinch more than an inch of fat, excluding muscles, chances are you have too much body fat.

Energy Balance and Counting Calories: Losing weight boils down to a simple mathematical formula: consume fewer calories than you burn. Learn how to balance energy intake (food) with energy output (calories burned by physical activity). If you take in more calories than your body needs to perform your day's activities, it will be stored as fat. Therefore, the only solution is to consume the proper amount of calories that your body needs to maintain good health. Then exercise so your body can utilize the stored fat. The end result will be your desired weight-loss.

CALORIES BURNED FOR PHYSICAL ACTIVITIES

LIGHT ACTIVITIES - 150 or less	CAL/HR.
Billiards	140
Lying down/sleeping	60
Office work	140
Sitting	80
Standing	100

MODERATE ACTIVITIES - 150-350	CAL/HR.
Aerobic Dancing	340
Ballroom dancing	210
Bicycling (5 mph)	170
Bowling	160
Canoeing (2.5 mph)	170
Dancing (social)	210
Gardening (moderate)	270
Golf (with cart)	180
Golf (without cart)	320
Grocery shopping	180
Horseback riding (sitting trot)	250
Light housework/cleaning, etc.	250
Ping pong	270
Swimming (20 yards/min)	290
Tennis (recreational doubles)	310
Vacuuming	220
Volleyball (recreational)	260
Walking (2 mph)	200
Walking (3 mph)	240
Walking (4 mph)	300

CALORIES BURNED FOR PHYSICAL ACTIVITIES

VIGOROUS ACTIVITIES - 350 or MORE	CAL/HR.
Aerobics (step)	440
Backpacking (10 lb load)	540
Badminton	450
Basketball (competitive)	660
Basketball (leisure)	390
Bicycling (10 mph)	375
Bicycling (13 mph)	600
Cross country skiing (leisurely)	460
Cross country skiing (moderate)	660
Hiking	460
Ice skating (9 mph)	384
Jogging (5 mph)	550
Jogging (6 mph)	690
Racquetball	620
Rollerblading	384
Rowing machine	540
Running (8 mph)	900
Scuba diving	570
Shoveling snow	580
Soccer	580
Spinning	650
Stair climber machine	480
Swimming (50 yards/min.)	680
Water aerobics	400
Water skiing	480
Weight training (30 sec. b/w sets)	760
Weight training (60 sec. b/w sets)	570

YOUR PERSONAL PROFILE

Begin your weight-loss program by completing some helpful information so you can assess your current physical state, habits, and eating patterns. This information will assist you in identifying the areas of your diet and health that need improvement.

Start out by completing statistics regarding your age, weight, height, body fat percentage, and Body Mass Index (see page 14). If you are a member of a gym, you can set up an appointment to get your body fat measured for a small fee. There are also scales available that will calculate your body fat percentage. Another option is purchasing an at home body fat analyzer, which is small hand-held device that measures your fat. These analyzers are affordable and can be purchased online or at your local health and fitness retailer.

Visit your primary care physician to find out important information regarding your health. Have your doctor measure your cholesterol, triglycerides, blood pressure and glucose levels. You can also check with your local drug store and see if the pharmacy offers this service for a nominal fee. This information will help you determine if you are at risk for certain diseases or conditions. In addition, these levels will also factor into the food choices you make when creating your diet. For example, if you have high blood pressure, you may want to reduce your sodium intake. Therefore, you should try to avoid foods with added salt. High levels of cholesterol and triglycerides (over 160 mg/dL for cholesterol, over 200 mg/dL for triglycerides) can put you at risk for heart related diseases. In this instance, you should limit the amount of saturated fats, trans fats and dietary cholesterol found in high fat dairy and meat products.

Finally, assess your current eating and physical habits. Document the types of foods you currently eat, when you typically have meals, and any other dietary requirements that you have. If you are active, write down the exercises you participate in and how often you do them. You can also answer some additional questions to help you define problem areas and assist you in determining the weight-loss plan that is most beneficial for your needs.

Complete the following personal health profile. You can request necessary information from your primary health care provider.

Name: _____   Total Cholesterol: _____

Age: _____   Triglycerides: _____

Weight: _____   HDL Cholesterol: _____

Height: _____   LDL Cholesterol: _____

Body Fat Percentage: _____   Blood Pressure: _____

Body Mass Index*: _____   Glucose: _____

*Refer to page 17 to determine your BMI

Current Diet & Eating Habits: (vegetarian, low carb, snack often, compulsive eating, etc.)

_____

_____

_____

_____

Current Physical Activity: (sedentary, moderately active, very active) _____

_____

_____

_____

_____

Other Current Habits: (smoking, drinking, lack of sleep, etc.)_____

_____

_____

_____

_____

The following questions will assist you in developing your weight-loss program. When choosing a specific diet program, determining your strength and weaknesses will help you figure out what plan is right for you.

Which best describes your daily eating habits?

❏ 3 average meals
❏ Graze frequently
❏ One large meal/little else

What types of food do you crave the most?

❏ Meat/fish
❏ Fruit/vegetables
❏ Bread/cereals/rice
❏ Sweets

Do you typically eat out or prepare food for yourself?

❏ I usually cook my own food
❏ I eat out or have pre-made meals

What is your weight-loss goal?

❏ Lose 20 or more pounds
❏ Maintain weight
❏ Lose a little weight
❏ Improve health

What is your fitness goal?

❏ Decrease fat
❏ Gain muscle
❏ Improve strength

Describe your body type:

❏ Overweight
❏ Average
❏ Muscular

What length of plan would you want to consider?

❏ Less than 1 month
❏ 1-3 months
❏ 3-6 months
❏ 6 or more months

What particular event do you want to lose weight for (if any)?

_____

_____

_____

_____

When developing your weight-loss program and goals, be sure to take into account the answers that you have noted above. These answers will factor into your decision when choosing the program that would be most effective and best suit your needs.

YOUR PERSONAL WEIGHT-LOSS
GOALS, PLANS, & ACHIEVEMENTS

Once you have created a weight-loss goal, write down the specific program information in this section. This way, you can easily keep track of the daily requirements for your diet.

Record the specific number of daily calories your plan allows, as well as the total grams of fat, protein, carbohydrates, fiber, and ounces of water that you should consume.

Decide if you want to incorporate an exercise plan into your weight-loss program. If so, you can outline the activities that you would like to include in this section and schedule them into your routine.

You can also look forward to documenting your results. In the space indicated, write down your current measurements and your desired measurements. Once you have completed your program, you can fill in your final information and compare your end results to your original statistics.

Two sets of pages have been supplied so you can create up to two different plans. If you begin one plan and find that it does not work for you, use the additional pages to outline a new goal and plan and include the adjustments that you need to make.

YOUR PERSONAL GOALS, PLANS, ACHIEVEMENTS

NAME OF PLAN: _____   START DATE: _____

LENGTH OF PLAN: _____   END DATE: _____

1.) DESCRIPTION OF GOAL

_____

_____

_____

_____

2.) DESCRIPTION OF DIET PLAN

_____

_____

_____

Depending on the amount of calories allotted daily per your diet, list below the daily targets that you would like to meet each day:

TOTAL DAILY CALORIES: _____

    Fat grams: _____   Carb grams: _____

    Protein grams: _____   Fiber grams: _____

    Water (oz.): _____   Other: _____

3.) DESCRIPTION OF EXERCISE PLAN

_____

_____

_____

If you are also including a fitness program into your plan, you can outline the activities that you would like to accomplish for each day of the week:

Mon: _____   Thurs: _____

Tues: _____   Fri: _____

Wed: _____   Sat/Sun: _____

4.) RESULTS

STATISTICS	BEFORE	DESIRED	AFTER
Weight			
Body Fat %			
Body Mass Index			
Chest			
Waist			
Hips			
Thigh			
Bicep			

BEFORE AND AFTER PHOTOS:

Be proud of your results! Take a "before" and "after" photo and paste them here so you can compare and track your progress:

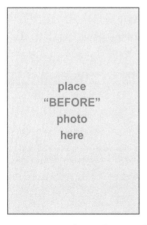

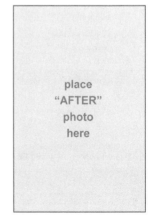

YOUR PERSONAL GOALS, PLANS, ACHIEVEMENTS

NAME OF PLAN: _____   START DATE: _____

LENGTH OF PLAN: _____   END DATE: _____

1.) DESCRIPTION OF GOAL

_____

_____

_____

_____

2.) DESCRIPTION OF DIET PLAN

_____

_____

_____

Depending on the amount of calories allotted daily per your diet, list below the daily targets that you would like to meet each day:

TOTAL DAILY CALORIES: _____

    Fat grams:_____   Carb grams: _____

    Protein grams: _____   Fiber grams:_____

    Water (oz.): _____   Other: _____

3.) DESCRIPTION OF EXERCISE PLAN

_____

_____

_____

If you are also including a fitness program into your plan, you can outline the activities that you would like to accomplish for each day of the week:

Mon:_____   Thurs:_____

Tues:_____   Fri: _____

Wed: _____   Sat/Sun: _____

4.) RESULTS

STATISTICS	BEFORE	DESIRED	AFTER
Weight			
Body Fat %			
Body Mass Index			
Chest			
Waist			
Hips			
Thigh			
Bicep			

BEFORE AND AFTER PHOTOS:

Be proud of your results! Take a "before" and "after" photo and paste them here so you can compare and track your progress:

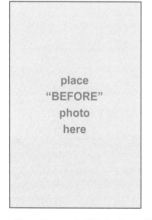

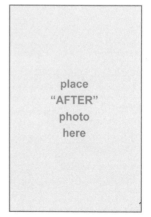

THE SECRET TO WEIGHT-LOSS:

KEEPING TRACK OF WHAT YOU EAT

For human weight, one pound of fat is equal to 3,500 stored calories. If weight-loss is viewed in the most simplistic of terms, it can be determined as the amount of calories consumed versus the amount of calories burned. If you burn more calories than you eat, then ideally you should lose weight.

The most important aspect of weight-loss is to be aware of how much food and the total number of calories you consume on a daily basis. This awareness can be created through the use of this diet journal. Why is it important to keep track of what you eat? By actively documenting the foods and beverages you consume on a daily basis, you are establishing the following criteria that will help you lose-weight.

Awareness: Keeping a diet journal builds your daily food awareness. Instead of mindlessly consuming meals, this diet journal will help you become conscious of what you are eating, how much, and how often. This awareness will help you realize that maybe you don't need as much food as you are currently eating. Perhaps you can be perfectly satisfied with less. With the use of this journal, you can discover how foods can affect your body. Do you feel sluggish after eating too many fatty foods? Do you feel energetic and refreshed after eating a salad and lean protein? You will also learn what foods have more calories, fat and nutrients than others. If you are aware of what your body needs to lose weight, you can make better, more informed food choices.

Reality: Many dieters do not realize how many calories are included in the foods that they consume. This diet journal allows you to break down your meals into total calories. At the end of each day, you can add up your daily totals. Then you can check and see if you have stayed within the range of calories suggested for your diet. For example, if you have a turkey and swiss bagel with mayo, a bag of chips, a chocolate chip cookie, and a soda for lunch, the calories versus a turkey pita with veggies, popcorn, and yogurt would be twice as much. Below are the approximate caloric values for both meals.

TURKEY SWISS BAGEL LUNCH	
370	large gourmet deli bagel
90	3 slices of 1 oz. turkey breast
220	2 1 oz. slices of swiss cheese
100	1 tbsp mayo
275	deli chocolate chip cookie
150	1 oz. snack bag chips
150	12 oz. can soda

1,355 TOTAL CALORIES
(approx.)

TURKEY PITA LUNCH	
170	whole wheat pita
90	3 slices of 1 oz. turkey breast
25	1 tbsp grated parmesan cheese
5	1 tsp mustard
20	veggies
60	2 cups light microwave popcorn
120	6 oz. non-fat flavored yogurt
0	water with lemon

435 TOTAL CALORIES
(approx.)

Once you realize where the majority of calories are coming from, you can make healthier, low calorie changes and eliminate the excess foods that do not have significant nutritional value. Some foods just have more calories than others. When you realize that an average blueberry scone from your local coffee shop has 450 calories and 17 grams of fat, you may want to choose an alternate breakfast of a whole wheat english muffin, an omelet with 2 egg whites, a 1 oz. slice of ham, tomatoes, onions, bell peppers and a medium banana for 340 calories and 6 grams of fat.

Accountability: Keeping a diet journal forces individuals to account for all food and beverages consumed on a daily basis. Many individuals who are seeking to lose weight allow hidden calories to sneak into their diet. By writing down all of the foods you eat and calculating the daily calorie and nutritional value for all your meals, you are forced to consider how an extra serving of pasta or a dessert will factor into your diet. Many people do not take into consideration their beverages when on a weight-loss program. If you favor whole milk lattés, smoothies, soda, alcoholic drinks, and juices, it is possible to drink as many calories as you get from your food. Be sure to include calories from all beverages, as well as solid food, and then determine whether or not you need to cut back.

Routine: When you start a diet journal, you establish a routine. This routine helps you to maintain a stable, steady progress towards your weight-loss goal. If you have a plan that you can count on for every day of the week, you are more likely to keep with your diet and avoid situations that can sabotage your diet. Even if you end up having a large meal with drinks and dessert, you have the benefit of having a solid foundation to which you can return the next day.

HOW TO START

Start out each day by assigning a two-page spread for the current date. Invest in a weight scale so you can accurately measure your weight-loss progress. Weigh yourself unclothed when you wake up in the morning, before breakfast, so you can get a fresh reading for the day. Write down this number at the top of the page. Gradually, as you make your progress, you will see this number move closer to your goal. Do not to worry if during your program, this number fluctuates up or down. There are many factors, such as water and muscle gain, that can affect your weight. A typical fluctuation can range from 2-3 pounds.

Daily Nutritional Intake: Begin by writing down all of the foods that you eat on a daily basis. The daily nutritional intake section is separated into 3 meals: breakfast, lunch, and dinner, as well as a fourth section for snacks. Write down the time you consume each meal, as well as all the items in your meal, including dressing, condiments, and beverages. To accurately assess your daily totals, it is extremely important to include all the items and the quantity of each.

Each meal has a section for comments. You can jot helpful information in this space that will assist you in planning or calculating your daily menu. For example, if you know you are going out to lunch at a restaurant, jot down several healthy menu options that would work with your diet plan.

Calories and Nutritional Values: For each meal, calculate your nutritional totals for calories, fat, carbohydrates, protein, and fiber. You can find the values for the most popular food items in the nutritional information section located in the back of this journal. This type of information can also be found online, or you can purchase a calorie counting book at your local bookstore. In addition, you can refer to the nutrition facts label printed on the container of most pre-packaged foods. Once you have made all of your documentation for the day, use the Daily Totals section to calculate the total number of calories you have consumed. Compare your totals to the number of calories suggested for your program. If you are at your target or under, you are on the right track. If you are a little over, do not worry. Just make some adjustments to your diet and try to choose more low-calorie options.

Exercise and Fitness: This section will encourage you to participate in physical activities on a daily basis. All types of physical activities burn calories so be sure to write down your exercise routine, the length of the session, and the approximate calories utilized by your body. This information can help you recognize your behaviors or habits that may lead to a successful weight-loss journey. It is also a source of reference to help you maintain your ideal body weight in the future.

Weight-loss is determined by the amount of calories consumed versus the amount burned. If you happen to have a "bad eating" day, you can try to make up for the excess calories by adding an additional exercise routine the following day. Since you will be completing this section on a daily basis, motivate yourself by incorporating the activities that you enjoy the most.

Energy Levels: Determine the relationship that your body has with food. Take notice of how your body responds to your weight-loss program. Document your daily overall energy levels at the bottom of the second page. See how your energy correlates to the types of foods you have included in your program. If you notice that a little extra protein helps you get through your workout, incorporate lean meats in your diet. As you discover these relationships, make adjustments as needed to help you feel your best.

Water Intake: Strive for a total of 8 eight-ounce glasses of water per day. Write down your daily intake to reach your healthy hydration goals. Many times people believe that they are hungry when they are actually thirsty. If you drink water on a normal basis throughout the day, you can maintain a constant level of hydration.

Vitamins and Supplements: This section is a great daily reminder if you are incorporating additional nutrients into your diet program. If you are restricting your daily caloric intake, it can be a good idea to take vitamins and supplements. If you choose to do so, mark it in your journal and be sure to keep track on a daily basis. You can also assess the effectiveness of your supplements over time by comparing your energy levels to the vitamins that you have taken. Also, if you make changes to food that you eat while on your diet, you may want to consider adapting your supplements as well. When in doubt about specific vitamin recommendations, consult with health care professionals.

Daily Goals Achieved: This is a quick way to track your daily progress towards your goal. If for any reason you did not meet your daily goal, reflect on the factors that kept you from your goal write them down. You can then decide on any changes that you can make to your diet or fitness plan to help you stay on track. Incorporate these improvements into your following day.

Daily Nutritional Intake
FOOD AND BEVERAGES

1/4

DATE   WEIGHT

MORNING/TIME:	cal.	fat	protein	carbs.	fiber
Coffee					
Cherries					
cinamon bear					
BREAKFAST TOTALS					

AFTERNOON/TIME:	cal.	fat	protein	carbs.	fiber
LUNCH TOTALS					

EVENING/TIME:	cal.	fat	protein	carbs.	fiber
DINNER TOTALS					

Daily Nutritional Intake
FOOD AND BEVERAGES

SNACKS/TIME:	cal.	fat	protein	carbs.	fiber
SNACK TOTALS					

	cal.	fat	protein	carbs.	fiber
DAILY TOTALS					

Exercise and Fitness
DAILY PHYSICAL ACTIVITIES

ACTIVITY	cal. burned
TOTAL CAL. BURNED	

Vitamins/Supplements
DAILY INTAKE

DESCRIPTION	qty/time

ENERGY LEVELS ❑ low ❑ med ❑ high   WATER #OZ. _____

57

Daily Nutritional Intake

FOOD AND BEVERAGES   DATE   WEIGHT

MORNING/TIME:	cal.	fat	protein	carbs.	fiber
BREAKFAST TOTALS					

AFTERNOON/TIME:	cal.	fat	protein	carbs.	fiber
LUNCH TOTALS					

EVENING/TIME:	cal.	fat	protein	carbs.	fiber
DINNER TOTALS					

Daily Nutritional Intake
FOOD AND BEVERAGES

DAILY GOALS ACHIEVED

SNACKS/TIME:	cal.	fat	protein	carbs.	fiber
SNACK TOTALS					

	cal.	fat	protein	carbs.	fiber
DAILY TOTALS					

Exercise and Fitness
DAILY PHYSICAL ACTIVITIES

ACTIVITY	cal. burned
TOTAL CAL. BURNED	

Vitamins/Supplements
DAILY INTAKE

DESCRIPTION	qty/time

ENERGY LEVELS ❑ low ❑ med ❑ high   WATER #OZ. _____

Daily Nutritional Intake
FOOD AND BEVERAGES   DATE   WEIGHT

MORNING/TIME:	cal.	fat	protein	carbs.	fiber
BREAKFAST TOTALS					

AFTERNOON/TIME:	cal.	fat	protein	carbs.	fiber
LUNCH TOTALS					

EVENING/TIME:	cal.	fat	protein	carbs.	fiber
DINNER TOTALS					

Daily Nutritional Intake
FOOD AND BEVERAGES

SNACKS/TIME:	cal.	fat	protein	carbs.	fiber
SNACK TOTALS					

	cal.	fat	protein	carbs.	fiber
DAILY TOTALS					

Exercise and Fitness
DAILY PHYSICAL ACTIVITIES

ACTIVITY	cal. burned
TOTAL CAL. BURNED	

Vitamins/Supplements
DAILY INTAKE

DESCRIPTION	qty/time

ENERGY LEVELS ❑ low ❑ med ❑ high   WATER #OZ. _____

_____

_____

_____

_____

Daily Nutritional Intake

FOOD AND BEVERAGES

DATE _____ WEIGHT _____

MORNING/TIME:	cal.	fat	protein	carbs.	fiber
BREAKFAST TOTALS					

AFTERNOON/TIME:	cal.	fat	protein	carbs.	fiber
LUNCH TOTALS					

EVENING/TIME:	cal.	fat	protein	carbs.	fiber
DINNER TOTALS					

Daily Nutritional Intake
FOOD AND BEVERAGES

SNACKS/TIME:	cal.	fat	protein	carbs.	fiber
SNACK TOTALS					

	cal.	fat	protein	carbs.	fiber
DAILY TOTALS					

Exercise and Fitness
DAILY PHYSICAL ACTIVITIES

ACTIVITY	cal. burned
TOTAL CAL. BURNED	

Vitamins/Supplements
DAILY INTAKE

DESCRIPTION	qty/time

ENERGY LEVELS ❑ low ❑ med ❑ high   **WATER #OZ.** _____

63

Daily Nutritional Intake

FOOD AND BEVERAGES

DATE   WEIGHT

MORNING/TIME:	cal.	fat	protein	carbs.	fiber
BREAKFAST TOTALS					

AFTERNOON/TIME:	cal.	fat	protein	carbs.	fiber
LUNCH TOTALS					

EVENING/TIME:	cal.	fat	protein	carbs.	fiber
DINNER TOTALS					

Daily Nutritional Intake
FOOD AND BEVERAGES

DAILY
GOALS
ACHIEVED

SNACKS/TIME:	cal.	fat	protein	carbs.	fiber
SNACK TOTALS					

	cal.	fat	protein	carbs.	fiber
DAILY TOTALS					

Exercise and Fitness
DAILY PHYSICAL ACTIVITIES

ACTIVITY	cal. burned
TOTAL CAL. BURNED	

Vitamins/Supplements
DAILY INTAKE

DESCRIPTION	qty/time

ENERGY LEVELS ❑ low ❑ med ❑ high   WATER #OZ. _____

Daily Nutritional Intake

FOOD AND BEVERAGES

DATE _____   WEIGHT _____

MORNING/TIME:	cal.	fat	protein	carbs.	fiber
BREAKFAST TOTALS					

AFTERNOON/TIME:	cal.	fat	protein	carbs.	fiber
LUNCH TOTALS					

EVENING/TIME:	cal.	fat	protein	carbs.	fiber
DINNER TOTALS					

Daily Nutritional Intake
FOOD AND BEVERAGES

SNACKS/TIME:	cal.	fat	protein	carbs.	fiber
SNACK TOTALS					

	cal.	fat	protein	carbs.	fiber
DAILY TOTALS					

Exercise and Fitness
DAILY PHYSICAL ACTIVITIES

ACTIVITY	cal. burned
TOTAL CAL. BURNED	

Vitamins/Supplements
DAILY INTAKE

DESCRIPTION	qty/time

ENERGY LEVELS ❑ low   ❑ med   ❑ high   WATER #OZ. _____

Daily Nutritional Intake

FOOD AND BEVERAGES

DATE   WEIGHT

MORNING/TIME:	cal.	fat	protein	carbs.	fiber
BREAKFAST TOTALS					

AFTERNOON/TIME:	cal.	fat	protein	carbs.	fiber
LUNCH TOTALS					

EVENING/TIME:	cal.	fat	protein	carbs.	fiber
DINNER TOTALS					

Daily Nutritional Intake
FOOD AND BEVERAGES

SNACKS/TIME:	cal.	fat	protein	carbs.	fiber
SNACK TOTALS					

	cal.	fat	protein	carbs.	fiber
DAILY TOTALS					

Exercise and Fitness
DAILY PHYSICAL ACTIVITIES

ACTIVITY	cal. burned
TOTAL CAL. BURNED	

Vitamins/Supplements
DAILY INTAKE

DESCRIPTION	qty/time

ENERGY LEVELS ❑ low ❑ med ❑ high   WATER #OZ. _____

_____

_____

_____

_____

69

Daily Nutritional Intake

FOOD AND BEVERAGES   DATE   WEIGHT

MORNING/TIME:	cal.	fat	protein	carbs.	fiber
BREAKFAST TOTALS					

AFTERNOON/TIME:	cal.	fat	protein	carbs.	fiber
LUNCH TOTALS					

EVENING/TIME:	cal.	fat	protein	carbs.	fiber
DINNER TOTALS					

Daily Nutritional Intake
FOOD AND BEVERAGES

DAILY
GOALS
ACHIEVED

SNACKS/TIME:	cal.	fat	protein	carbs.	fiber
SNACK TOTALS					

	cal.	fat	protein	carbs.	fiber
DAILY TOTALS					

Exercise and Fitness
DAILY PHYSICAL ACTIVITIES

ACTIVITY	cal. burned
TOTAL CAL. BURNED	

Vitamins/Supplements
DAILY INTAKE

DESCRIPTION	qty/time

ENERGY LEVELS ❑ low ❑ med ❑ high   WATER #OZ. _____

_____
_____
_____
_____

Daily Nutritional Intake

FOOD AND BEVERAGES

DATE _____ WEIGHT _____

MORNING/TIME:	cal.	fat	protein	carbs.	fiber
BREAKFAST TOTALS					

AFTERNOON/TIME:	cal.	fat	protein	carbs.	fiber
LUNCH TOTALS					

EVENING/TIME:	cal.	fat	protein	carbs.	fiber
DINNER TOTALS					

Daily Nutritional Intake
FOOD AND BEVERAGES

SNACKS/TIME:	cal.	fat	protein	carbs.	fiber
SNACK TOTALS					

	cal.	fat	protein	carbs.	fiber
DAILY TOTALS					

Exercise and Fitness
DAILY PHYSICAL ACTIVITIES

ACTIVITY	cal. burned
TOTAL CAL. BURNED	

Vitamins/Supplements
DAILY INTAKE

DESCRIPTION	qty/time

ENERGY LEVELS ❑ low ❑ med ❑ high   **WATER #OZ.** _____

Daily Nutritional Intake

FOOD AND BEVERAGES

DATE   WEIGHT

MORNING/TIME:	cal.	fat	protein	carbs.	fiber
BREAKFAST TOTALS					

AFTERNOON/TIME:	cal.	fat	protein	carbs.	fiber
LUNCH TOTALS					

EVENING/TIME:	cal.	fat	protein	carbs.	fiber
DINNER TOTALS					

Daily Nutritional Intake
FOOD AND BEVERAGES

DAILY
GOALS
ACHIEVED

SNACKS/TIME:	cal.	fat	protein	carbs.	fiber
SNACK TOTALS					

	cal.	fat	protein	carbs.	fiber
DAILY TOTALS					

Exercise and Fitness
DAILY PHYSICAL ACTIVITIES

ACTIVITY	cal. burned
TOTAL CAL. BURNED	

Vitamins/Supplements
DAILY INTAKE

DESCRIPTION	qty/time

ENERGY LEVELS ❑ low ❑ med ❑ high   WATER #OZ. _____

_____
_____
_____
_____

Daily Nutritional Intake

FOOD AND BEVERAGES | DATE | WEIGHT

MORNING/TIME:	cal.	fat	protein	carbs.	fiber
BREAKFAST TOTALS					

AFTERNOON/TIME:	cal.	fat	protein	carbs.	fiber
LUNCH TOTALS					

EVENING/TIME:	cal.	fat	protein	carbs.	fiber
DINNER TOTALS					

Daily Nutritional Intake
FOOD AND BEVERAGES

DAILY GOALS ACHIEVED

SNACKS/TIME:	cal.	fat	protein	carbs.	fiber
SNACK TOTALS					

	cal.	fat	protein	carbs.	fiber
DAILY TOTALS					

Exercise and Fitness
DAILY PHYSICAL ACTIVITIES

ACTIVITY	cal. burned
TOTAL CAL. BURNED	

Vitamins/Supplements
DAILY INTAKE

DESCRIPTION	qty/time

ENERGY LEVELS ❏ low ❏ med ❏ high   WATER #OZ. _____

Daily Nutritional Intake

FOOD AND BEVERAGES

DATE   WEIGHT

MORNING/TIME:	cal.	fat	protein	carbs.	fiber
BREAKFAST TOTALS					

AFTERNOON/TIME:	cal.	fat	protein	carbs.	fiber
LUNCH TOTALS					

EVENING/TIME:	cal.	fat	protein	carbs.	fiber
DINNER TOTALS					

Daily Nutritional Intake
FOOD AND BEVERAGES

DAILY GOALS ACHIEVED

SNACKS/TIME:	cal.	fat	protein	carbs.	fiber
SNACK TOTALS					

	cal.	fat	protein	carbs.	fiber
DAILY TOTALS					

Exercise and Fitness
DAILY PHYSICAL ACTIVITIES

ACTIVITY	cal. burned
TOTAL CAL. BURNED	

Vitamins/Supplements
DAILY INTAKE

DESCRIPTION	qty/time

ENERGY LEVELS ☐ low ☐ med ☐ high   WATER #OZ. _____

Daily Nutritional Intake

FOOD AND BEVERAGES   DATE   WEIGHT

MORNING/TIME:	cal.	fat	protein	carbs.	fiber
BREAKFAST TOTALS					

AFTERNOON/TIME:	cal.	fat	protein	carbs.	fiber
LUNCH TOTALS					

EVENING/TIME:	cal.	fat	protein	carbs.	fiber
DINNER TOTALS					

Daily Nutritional Intake
FOOD AND BEVERAGES

SNACKS/TIME:	cal.	fat	protein	carbs.	fiber
SNACK TOTALS					

	cal.	fat	protein	carbs.	fiber
DAILY TOTALS					

Exercise and Fitness
DAILY PHYSICAL ACTIVITIES

ACTIVITY	cal. burned
TOTAL CAL. BURNED	

Vitamins/Supplements
DAILY INTAKE

DESCRIPTION	qty/time

ENERGY LEVELS ☐ low ☐ med ☐ high   WATER #OZ. _____

_____

_____

_____

81

Daily Nutritional Intake

FOOD AND BEVERAGES

DATE _____ WEIGHT _____

MORNING/TIME:	cal.	fat	protein	carbs.	fiber
BREAKFAST TOTALS					

AFTERNOON/TIME:	cal.	fat	protein	carbs.	fiber
LUNCH TOTALS					

EVENING/TIME:	cal.	fat	protein	carbs.	fiber
DINNER TOTALS					

Daily Nutritional Intake
FOOD AND BEVERAGES

DAILY
GOALS
ACHIEVED I DID IT!

SNACKS/TIME:	cal.	fat	protein	carbs.	fiber
SNACK TOTALS					

	cal.	fat	protein	carbs.	fiber
DAILY TOTALS					

Exercise and Fitness
DAILY PHYSICAL ACTIVITIES

ACTIVITY	cal. burned
TOTAL CAL. BURNED	

Vitamins/Supplements
DAILY INTAKE

DESCRIPTION	qty/time

ENERGY LEVELS ❑ low ❑ med ❑ high   WATER #OZ. _____

Daily Nutritional Intake
FOOD AND BEVERAGES

DATE   WEIGHT

MORNING/TIME:	cal.	fat	protein	carbs.	fiber
BREAKFAST TOTALS					

AFTERNOON/TIME:	cal.	fat	protein	carbs.	fiber
LUNCH TOTALS					

EVENING/TIME:	cal.	fat	protein	carbs.	fiber
DINNER TOTALS					

Daily Nutritional Intake
FOOD AND BEVERAGES

SNACKS/TIME:	cal.	fat	protein	carbs.	fiber
SNACK TOTALS					

	cal.	fat	protein	carbs.	fiber
DAILY TOTALS					

Exercise and Fitness
DAILY PHYSICAL ACTIVITIES

ACTIVITY	cal. burned
TOTAL CAL. BURNED	

Vitamins/Supplements
DAILY INTAKE

DESCRIPTION	qty/time

ENERGY LEVELS ❑ low ❑ med ❑ high   WATER #OZ. _____

85

Daily Nutritional Intake

FOOD AND BEVERAGES   DATE   WEIGHT

MORNING/TIME:	cal.	fat	protein	carbs.	fiber
BREAKFAST TOTALS					

AFTERNOON/TIME:	cal.	fat	protein	carbs.	fiber
LUNCH TOTALS					

EVENING/TIME:	cal.	fat	protein	carbs.	fiber
DINNER TOTALS					

Daily Nutritional Intake

FOOD AND BEVERAGES

DAILY
GOALS
ACHIEVED I DID IT!

SNACKS/TIME:	cal.	fat	protein	carbs.	fiber
SNACK TOTALS					

	cal.	fat	protein	carbs.	fiber
DAILY TOTALS					

Exercise and Fitness

DAILY PHYSICAL ACTIVITIES

ACTIVITY	cal. burned
TOTAL CAL. BURNED	

Vitamins/Supplements

DAILY INTAKE

DESCRIPTION	qty/time

ENERGY LEVELS ☐ low ☐ med ☐ high   **WATER #OZ.** _____

Daily Nutritional Intake

FOOD AND BEVERAGES   DATE   WEIGHT

MORNING/TIME:	cal.	fat	protein	carbs.	fiber
BREAKFAST TOTALS					

AFTERNOON/TIME:	cal.	fat	protein	carbs.	fiber
LUNCH TOTALS					

EVENING/TIME:	cal.	fat	protein	carbs.	fiber
DINNER TOTALS					

Daily Nutritional Intake
FOOD AND BEVERAGES

SNACKS/TIME:	cal.	fat	protein	carbs.	fiber
SNACK TOTALS					

	cal.	fat	protein	carbs.	fiber
DAILY TOTALS					

Exercise and Fitness
DAILY PHYSICAL ACTIVITIES

ACTIVITY	cal. burned
TOTAL CAL. BURNED	

Vitamins/Supplements
DAILY INTAKE

DESCRIPTION	qty/time

ENERGY LEVELS ☐ low ☐ med ☐ high   **WATER #OZ.** _____

Daily Nutritional Intake

FOOD AND BEVERAGES

DATE   WEIGHT

MORNING/TIME:	cal.	fat	protein	carbs.	fiber
BREAKFAST TOTALS					

AFTERNOON/TIME:	cal.	fat	protein	carbs.	fiber
LUNCH TOTALS					

EVENING/TIME:	cal.	fat	protein	carbs.	fiber
DINNER TOTALS					

Daily Nutritional Intake

FOOD AND BEVERAGES

DAILY
GOALS
ACHIEVED

SNACKS/TIME:	cal.	fat	protein	carbs.	fiber
SNACK TOTALS					

	cal.	fat	protein	carbs.	fiber
DAILY TOTALS					

Exercise and Fitness

DAILY PHYSICAL ACTIVITIES

ACTIVITY	cal. burned
TOTAL CAL. BURNED	

Vitamins/Supplements

DAILY INTAKE

DESCRIPTION	qty/time

ENERGY LEVELS ❑ low ❑ med ❑ high   WATER #OZ. _____

_____

_____

_____

_____

Daily Nutritional Intake
FOOD AND BEVERAGES

DATE _____ WEIGHT _____

MORNING/TIME:	cal.	fat	protein	carbs.	fiber
BREAKFAST TOTALS					

AFTERNOON/TIME:	cal.	fat	protein	carbs.	fiber
LUNCH TOTALS					

EVENING/TIME:	cal.	fat	protein	carbs.	fiber
DINNER TOTALS					

Daily Nutritional Intake
FOOD AND BEVERAGES

DAILY GOALS ACHIEVED

SNACKS/TIME:	cal.	fat	protein	carbs.	fiber
SNACK TOTALS					

	cal.	fat	protein	carbs.	fiber
DAILY TOTALS					

Exercise and Fitness
DAILY PHYSICAL ACTIVITIES

ACTIVITY	cal. burned
TOTAL CAL. BURNED	

Vitamins/Supplements
DAILY INTAKE

DESCRIPTION	qty/time

ENERGY LEVELS ❑ low ❑ med ❑ high   WATER #OZ. _____

Daily Nutritional Intake

FOOD AND BEVERAGES

DATE _____   WEIGHT _____

MORNING/TIME:	cal.	fat	protein	carbs.	fiber
BREAKFAST TOTALS					

AFTERNOON/TIME:	cal.	fat	protein	carbs.	fiber
LUNCH TOTALS					

EVENING/TIME:	cal.	fat	protein	carbs.	fiber
DINNER TOTALS					

Daily Nutritional Intake
FOOD AND BEVERAGES

DAILY
GOALS
ACHIEVED

I DID IT!

SNACKS/TIME:	cal.	fat	protein	carbs.	fiber
SNACK TOTALS					

	cal.	fat	protein	carbs.	fiber
DAILY TOTALS					

Exercise and Fitness
DAILY PHYSICAL ACTIVITIES

ACTIVITY	cal. burned
TOTAL CAL. BURNED	

Vitamins/Supplements
DAILY INTAKE

DESCRIPTION	qty/time

ENERGY LEVELS ☐ low ☐ med ☐ high   WATER #OZ. _____

Daily Nutritional Intake

FOOD AND BEVERAGES

DATE   WEIGHT

MORNING/TIME:	cal.	fat	protein	carbs.	fiber
BREAKFAST TOTALS					

AFTERNOON/TIME:	cal.	fat	protein	carbs.	fiber
LUNCH TOTALS					

EVENING/TIME:	cal.	fat	protein	carbs.	fiber
DINNER TOTALS					

Daily Nutritional Intake
FOOD AND BEVERAGES

SNACKS/TIME:	cal.	fat	protein	carbs.	fiber
SNACK TOTALS					

	cal.	fat	protein	carbs.	fiber
DAILY TOTALS					

Exercise and Fitness
DAILY PHYSICAL ACTIVITIES

ACTIVITY	cal. burned
TOTAL CAL. BURNED	

Vitamins/Supplements
DAILY INTAKE

DESCRIPTION	qty/time

ENERGY LEVELS ❑ low ❑ med ❑ high   WATER #OZ. _____

Daily Nutritional Intake

FOOD AND BEVERAGES   DATE   WEIGHT

MORNING/TIME:	cal.	fat	protein	carbs.	fiber
BREAKFAST TOTALS					

AFTERNOON/TIME:	cal.	fat	protein	carbs.	fiber
LUNCH TOTALS					

EVENING/TIME:	cal.	fat	protein	carbs.	fiber
DINNER TOTALS					

Daily Nutritional Intake
FOOD AND BEVERAGES

SNACKS/TIME:	cal.	fat	protein	carbs.	fiber
SNACK TOTALS					

	cal.	fat	protein	carbs.	fiber
DAILY TOTALS					

Exercise and Fitness
DAILY PHYSICAL ACTIVITIES

ACTIVITY	cal. burned
TOTAL CAL. BURNED	

Vitamins/Supplements
DAILY INTAKE

DESCRIPTION	qty/time

ENERGY LEVELS ❏ low ❏ med ❏ high   WATER #OZ. _____

Daily Nutritional Intake

FOOD AND BEVERAGES   DATE   WEIGHT

MORNING/TIME:	cal.	fat	protein	carbs.	fiber
BREAKFAST TOTALS					

AFTERNOON/TIME:	cal.	fat	protein	carbs.	fiber
LUNCH TOTALS					

EVENING/TIME:	cal.	fat	protein	carbs.	fiber
DINNER TOTALS					

Daily Nutritional Intake
FOOD AND BEVERAGES

SNACKS/TIME:	cal.	fat	protein	carbs.	fiber
SNACK TOTALS					

	cal.	fat	protein	carbs.	fiber
DAILY TOTALS					

Exercise and Fitness
DAILY PHYSICAL ACTIVITIES

ACTIVITY	cal. burned
TOTAL CAL. BURNED	

Vitamins/Supplements
DAILY INTAKE

DESCRIPTION	qty/time

ENERGY LEVELS ❑ low ❑ med ❑ high   WATER #OZ. _____

_____

_____

_____

_____

Daily Nutritional Intake

FOOD AND BEVERAGES

DATE   WEIGHT

MORNING/TIME:	cal.	fat	protein	carbs.	fiber
BREAKFAST TOTALS					

AFTERNOON/TIME:	cal.	fat	protein	carbs.	fiber
LUNCH TOTALS					

EVENING/TIME:	cal.	fat	protein	carbs.	fiber
DINNER TOTALS					

Daily Nutritional Intake
FOOD AND BEVERAGES

SNACKS/TIME:	cal.	fat	protein	carbs.	fiber
SNACK TOTALS					

	cal.	fat	protein	carbs.	fiber
DAILY TOTALS					

Exercise and Fitness
DAILY PHYSICAL ACTIVITIES

ACTIVITY	cal. burned
TOTAL CAL. BURNED	

Vitamins/Supplements
DAILY INTAKE

DESCRIPTION	qty/time

ENERGY LEVELS ❑ low ❑ med ❑ high   WATER #OZ. _____

_____

_____

_____

_____

Daily Nutritional Intake

FOOD AND BEVERAGES

DATE   WEIGHT

MORNING/TIME:	cal.	fat	protein	carbs.	fiber
BREAKFAST TOTALS					

AFTERNOON/TIME:	cal.	fat	protein	carbs.	fiber
LUNCH TOTALS					

EVENING/TIME:	cal.	fat	protein	carbs.	fiber
DINNER TOTALS					

Daily Nutritional Intake
FOOD AND BEVERAGES

DAILY GOALS ACHIEVED

SNACKS/TIME:	cal.	fat	protein	carbs.	fiber
SNACK TOTALS					

	cal.	fat	protein	carbs.	fiber
DAILY TOTALS					

Exercise and Fitness
DAILY PHYSICAL ACTIVITIES

ACTIVITY	cal. burned
TOTAL CAL. BURNED	

Vitamins/Supplements
DAILY INTAKE

DESCRIPTION	qty/time

ENERGY LEVELS ☐ low ☐ med ☐ high   WATER #OZ. _____

Daily Nutritional Intake

FOOD AND BEVERAGES

DATE   WEIGHT

MORNING/TIME:	cal.	fat	protein	carbs.	fiber
BREAKFAST TOTALS					

AFTERNOON/TIME:	cal.	fat	protein	carbs.	fiber
LUNCH TOTALS					

EVENING/TIME:	cal.	fat	protein	carbs.	fiber
DINNER TOTALS					

Daily Nutritional Intake
FOOD AND BEVERAGES

SNACKS/TIME:	cal.	fat	protein	carbs.	fiber
SNACK TOTALS					

	cal.	fat	protein	carbs.	fiber
DAILY TOTALS					

Exercise and Fitness
DAILY PHYSICAL ACTIVITIES

ACTIVITY	cal. burned
TOTAL CAL. BURNED	

Vitamins/Supplements
DAILY INTAKE

DESCRIPTION	qty/time

ENERGY LEVELS ☐ low ☐ med ☐ high   WATER #OZ. _____

Daily Nutritional Intake

FOOD AND BEVERAGES   DATE   WEIGHT

MORNING/TIME:	cal.	fat	protein	carbs.	fiber
BREAKFAST TOTALS					

AFTERNOON/TIME:	cal.	fat	protein	carbs.	fiber
LUNCH TOTALS					

EVENING/TIME:	cal.	fat	protein	carbs.	fiber
DINNER TOTALS					

Daily Nutritional Intake
FOOD AND BEVERAGES

SNACKS/TIME:	cal.	fat	protein	carbs.	fiber
SNACK TOTALS					

	cal.	fat	protein	carbs.	fiber
DAILY TOTALS					

Exercise and Fitness
DAILY PHYSICAL ACTIVITIES

ACTIVITY	cal. burned
TOTAL CAL. BURNED	

Vitamins/Supplements
DAILY INTAKE

DESCRIPTION	qty/time

ENERGY LEVELS ❑ low ❑ med ❑ high   WATER #OZ. _____

Daily Nutritional Intake

FOOD AND BEVERAGES   DATE   WEIGHT

MORNING/TIME:	cal.	fat	protein	carbs.	fiber
BREAKFAST TOTALS					

AFTERNOON/TIME:	cal.	fat	protein	carbs.	fiber
LUNCH TOTALS					

EVENING/TIME:	cal.	fat	protein	carbs.	fiber
DINNER TOTALS					

Daily Nutritional Intake
FOOD AND BEVERAGES

SNACKS/TIME:	cal.	fat	protein	carbs.	fiber
SNACK TOTALS					

	cal.	fat	protein	carbs.	fiber
DAILY TOTALS					

Exercise and Fitness
DAILY PHYSICAL ACTIVITIES

ACTIVITY	cal. burned
TOTAL CAL. BURNED	

Vitamins/Supplements
DAILY INTAKE

DESCRIPTION	qty/time

ENERGY LEVELS ☐ low ☐ med ☐ high　　WATER #OZ. _____

Daily Nutritional Intake

FOOD AND BEVERAGES   DATE   WEIGHT

MORNING/TIME:	cal.	fat	protein	carbs.	fiber
BREAKFAST TOTALS					

AFTERNOON/TIME:	cal.	fat	protein	carbs.	fiber
LUNCH TOTALS					

EVENING/TIME:	cal.	fat	protein	carbs.	fiber
DINNER TOTALS					

Daily Nutritional Intake
FOOD AND BEVERAGES

DAILY
GOALS
ACHIEVED

SNACKS/TIME:	cal.	fat	protein	carbs.	fiber
SNACK TOTALS					

	cal.	fat	protein	carbs.	fiber
DAILY TOTALS					

Exercise and Fitness
DAILY PHYSICAL ACTIVITIES

ACTIVITY	cal. burned
TOTAL CAL. BURNED	

Vitamins/Supplements
DAILY INTAKE

DESCRIPTION	qty/time

ENERGY LEVELS ❑ low ❑ med ❑ high   WATER #oz. _____

_____

_____

_____

_____

Daily Nutritional Intake

FOOD AND BEVERAGES   DATE   WEIGHT

MORNING/TIME:	cal.	fat	protein	carbs.	fiber
BREAKFAST TOTALS					

AFTERNOON/TIME:	cal.	fat	protein	carbs.	fiber
LUNCH TOTALS					

EVENING/TIME:	cal.	fat	protein	carbs.	fiber
DINNER TOTALS					

Daily Nutritional Intake
FOOD AND BEVERAGES

SNACKS/TIME:	cal.	fat	protein	carbs.	fiber
SNACK TOTALS					

	cal.	fat	protein	carbs.	fiber
DAILY TOTALS					

Exercise and Fitness
DAILY PHYSICAL ACTIVITIES

ACTIVITY	cal. burned
TOTAL CAL. BURNED	

Vitamins/Supplements
DAILY INTAKE

DESCRIPTION	qty/time

ENERGY LEVELS ❑ low ❑ med ❑ high   WATER #OZ. _____

115

Daily Nutritional Intake

FOOD AND BEVERAGES　　　　　　　　　DATE　　　　WEIGHT

MORNING/TIME:	cal.	fat	protein	carbs.	fiber
BREAKFAST TOTALS					

AFTERNOON/TIME:	cal.	fat	protein	carbs.	fiber
LUNCH TOTALS					

EVENING/TIME:	cal.	fat	protein	carbs.	fiber
DINNER TOTALS					

Daily Nutritional Intake
FOOD AND BEVERAGES

DAILY
GOALS
ACHIEVED

SNACKS/TIME:	cal.	fat	protein	carbs.	fiber
SNACK TOTALS					

	cal.	fat	protein	carbs.	fiber
DAILY TOTALS					

Exercise and Fitness
DAILY PHYSICAL ACTIVITIES

ACTIVITY	cal. burned
TOTAL CAL. BURNED	

Vitamins/Supplements
DAILY INTAKE

DESCRIPTION	qty/time

ENERGY LEVELS ❑ low ❑ med ❑ high   WATER #OZ. _____

Daily Nutritional Intake
FOOD AND BEVERAGES   DATE   WEIGHT

MORNING/TIME:	cal.	fat	protein	carbs.	fiber
BREAKFAST TOTALS					

AFTERNOON/TIME:	cal.	fat	protein	carbs.	fiber
LUNCH TOTALS					

EVENING/TIME:	cal.	fat	protein	carbs.	fiber
DINNER TOTALS					

Daily Nutritional Intake
FOOD AND BEVERAGES

SNACKS/TIME:	cal.	fat	protein	carbs.	fiber
SNACK TOTALS					

	cal.	fat	protein	carbs.	fiber
DAILY TOTALS					

Exercise and Fitness
DAILY PHYSICAL ACTIVITIES

ACTIVITY	cal. burned
TOTAL CAL. BURNED	

Vitamins/Supplements
DAILY INTAKE

DESCRIPTION	qty/time

ENERGY LEVELS ❑ low ❑ med ❑ high   WATER #OZ. _____

Daily Nutritional Intake

FOOD AND BEVERAGES

DATE _____   WEIGHT _____

MORNING/TIME:	cal.	fat	protein	carbs.	fiber
BREAKFAST TOTALS					

AFTERNOON/TIME:	cal.	fat	protein	carbs.	fiber
LUNCH TOTALS					

EVENING/TIME:	cal.	fat	protein	carbs.	fiber
DINNER TOTALS					

Daily Nutritional Intake
FOOD AND BEVERAGES

DAILY
GOALS
ACHIEVED

SNACKS/TIME:	cal.	fat	protein	carbs.	fiber
SNACK TOTALS					

	cal.	fat	protein	carbs.	fiber
DAILY TOTALS					

Exercise and Fitness
DAILY PHYSICAL ACTIVITIES

ACTIVITY	cal. burned
TOTAL CAL. BURNED	

Vitamins/Supplements
DAILY INTAKE

DESCRIPTION	qty/time

ENERGY LEVELS ❑ low ❑ med ❑ high   WATER #OZ. _____

_____

_____

_____

_____

Daily Nutritional Intake
FOOD AND BEVERAGES

DATE   WEIGHT

MORNING/TIME:	cal.	fat	protein	carbs.	fiber
BREAKFAST TOTALS					

AFTERNOON/TIME:	cal.	fat	protein	carbs.	fiber
LUNCH TOTALS					

EVENING/TIME:	cal.	fat	protein	carbs.	fiber
DINNER TOTALS					

Daily Nutritional Intake
FOOD AND BEVERAGES

DAILY
GOALS
ACHIEVED

SNACKS/TIME:	cal.	fat	protein	carbs.	fiber
SNACK TOTALS					

	cal.	fat	protein	carbs.	fiber
DAILY TOTALS					

Exercise and Fitness
DAILY PHYSICAL ACTIVITIES

ACTIVITY	cal. burned
TOTAL CAL. BURNED	

Vitamins/Supplements
DAILY INTAKE

DESCRIPTION	qty/time
	.

ENERGY LEVELS ❑ low ❑ med ❑ high   WATER #OZ. _____

123

Daily Nutritional Intake

FOOD AND BEVERAGES

DATE   WEIGHT

MORNING/TIME:	cal.	fat	protein	carbs.	fiber
BREAKFAST TOTALS					

AFTERNOON/TIME:	cal.	fat	protein	carbs.	fiber
LUNCH TOTALS					

EVENING/TIME:	cal.	fat	protein	carbs.	fiber
DINNER TOTALS					

Daily Nutritional Intake
FOOD AND BEVERAGES

DAILY GOALS ACHIEVED I DID IT!

SNACKS/TIME:	cal.	fat	protein	carbs.	fiber
SNACK TOTALS					

	cal.	fat	protein	carbs.	fiber
DAILY TOTALS					

Exercise and Fitness
DAILY PHYSICAL ACTIVITIES

ACTIVITY	cal. burned
TOTAL CAL. BURNED	

Vitamins/Supplements
DAILY INTAKE

DESCRIPTION	qty/time

ENERGY LEVELS ❑ low ❑ med ❑ high   WATER #OZ. _____

Daily Nutritional Intake

FOOD AND BEVERAGES   DATE   WEIGHT

MORNING/TIME:	cal.	fat	protein	carbs.	fiber
BREAKFAST TOTALS					

AFTERNOON/TIME:	cal.	fat	protein	carbs.	fiber
LUNCH TOTALS					

EVENING/TIME:	cal.	fat	protein	carbs.	fiber
DINNER TOTALS					

Daily Nutritional Intake
FOOD AND BEVERAGES

SNACKS/TIME:	cal.	fat	protein	carbs.	fiber
SNACK TOTALS					

	cal.	fat	protein	carbs.	fiber
DAILY TOTALS					

Exercise and Fitness
DAILY PHYSICAL ACTIVITIES

ACTIVITY	cal. burned
TOTAL CAL. BURNED	

Vitamins/Supplements
DAILY INTAKE

DESCRIPTION	qty/time

ENERGY LEVELS ❑ low ❑ med ❑ high   WATER #OZ. _____

Daily Nutritional Intake

FOOD AND BEVERAGES   DATE   WEIGHT

MORNING/TIME:	cal.	fat	protein	carbs.	fiber
BREAKFAST TOTALS					

AFTERNOON/TIME:	cal.	fat	protein	carbs.	fiber
LUNCH TOTALS					

EVENING/TIME:	cal.	fat	protein	carbs.	fiber
DINNER TOTALS					

Daily Nutritional Intake
FOOD AND BEVERAGES

DAILY
GOALS
ACHIEVED

SNACKS/TIME:	cal.	fat	protein	carbs.	fiber
SNACK TOTALS					

	cal.	fat	protein	carbs.	fiber
DAILY TOTALS					

Exercise and Fitness
DAILY PHYSICAL ACTIVITIES

ACTIVITY	cal. burned
TOTAL CAL. BURNED	

Vitamins/Supplements
DAILY INTAKE

DESCRIPTION	qty/time

ENERGY LEVELS ☐ low ☐ med ☐ high   **WATER #OZ.** _____

Daily Nutritional Intake

FOOD AND BEVERAGES   DATE   WEIGHT

MORNING/TIME:	cal.	fat	protein	carbs.	fiber
BREAKFAST TOTALS					

AFTERNOON/TIME:	cal.	fat	protein	carbs.	fiber
LUNCH TOTALS					

EVENING/TIME:	cal.	fat	protein	carbs.	fiber
DINNER TOTALS					

Daily Nutritional Intake
FOOD AND BEVERAGES

SNACKS/TIME:	cal.	fat	protein	carbs.	fiber
SNACK TOTALS					

	cal.	fat	protein	carbs.	fiber
DAILY TOTALS					

Exercise and Fitness
DAILY PHYSICAL ACTIVITIES

ACTIVITY	cal. burned
TOTAL CAL. BURNED	

Vitamins/Supplements
DAILY INTAKE

DESCRIPTION	qty/time

ENERGY LEVELS ❑ low ❑ med ❑ high   WATER #OZ. _____

Daily Nutritional Intake

FOOD AND BEVERAGES

DATE   WEIGHT

MORNING/TIME:	cal.	fat	protein	carbs.	fiber
BREAKFAST TOTALS					

AFTERNOON/TIME:	cal.	fat	protein	carbs.	fiber
LUNCH TOTALS					

EVENING/TIME:	cal.	fat	protein	carbs.	fiber
DINNER TOTALS					

Daily Nutritional Intake
FOOD AND BEVERAGES

DAILY
GOALS
ACHIEVED

SNACKS/TIME:	cal.	fat	protein	carbs.	fiber
SNACK TOTALS					

	cal.	fat	protein	carbs.	fiber
DAILY TOTALS					

Exercise and Fitness
DAILY PHYSICAL ACTIVITIES

ACTIVITY	cal. burned
TOTAL CAL. BURNED	

Vitamins/Supplements
DAILY INTAKE

DESCRIPTION	qty/time

ENERGY LEVELS ❑ low ❑ med ❑ high   WATER #OZ. _____

133

Daily Nutritional Intake

FOOD AND BEVERAGES   DATE   WEIGHT

MORNING/TIME:	cal.	fat	protein	carbs.	fiber
BREAKFAST TOTALS					

AFTERNOON/TIME:	cal.	fat	protein	carbs.	fiber
LUNCH TOTALS					

EVENING/TIME:	cal.	fat	protein	carbs.	fiber
DINNER TOTALS					

Daily Nutritional Intake
FOOD AND BEVERAGES

SNACKS/TIME:	cal.	fat	protein	carbs.	fiber
SNACK TOTALS					

	cal.	fat	protein	carbs.	fiber
DAILY TOTALS					

Exercise and Fitness
DAILY PHYSICAL ACTIVITIES

ACTIVITY	cal. burned
TOTAL CAL. BURNED	

Vitamins/Supplements
DAILY INTAKE

DESCRIPTION	qty/time

ENERGY LEVELS ❑ low ❑ med ❑ high   WATER #OZ. _____

Daily Nutritional Intake

FOOD AND BEVERAGES — DATE — WEIGHT

MORNING/TIME:	cal.	fat	protein	carbs.	fiber
BREAKFAST TOTALS					

AFTERNOON/TIME:	cal.	fat	protein	carbs.	fiber
LUNCH TOTALS					

EVENING/TIME:	cal.	fat	protein	carbs.	fiber
DINNER TOTALS					

Daily Nutritional Intake
FOOD AND BEVERAGES

SNACKS/TIME:	cal.	fat	protein	carbs.	fiber
SNACK TOTALS					

	cal.	fat	protein	carbs.	fiber
DAILY TOTALS					

Exercise and Fitness
DAILY PHYSICAL ACTIVITIES

ACTIVITY	cal. burned
TOTAL CAL. BURNED	

Vitamins/Supplements
DAILY INTAKE

DESCRIPTION	qty/time

ENERGY LEVELS ❑ low ❑ med ❑ high   WATER #OZ. _____

137

Daily Nutritional Intake

FOOD AND BEVERAGES   DATE   WEIGHT

MORNING/TIME:	cal.	fat	protein	carbs.	fiber
BREAKFAST TOTALS					

AFTERNOON/TIME:	cal.	fat	protein	carbs.	fiber
LUNCH TOTALS					

EVENING/TIME:	cal.	fat	protein	carbs.	fiber
DINNER TOTALS					

Daily Nutritional Intake
FOOD AND BEVERAGES

SNACKS/TIME:	cal.	fat	protein	carbs.	fiber
SNACK TOTALS					

	cal.	fat	protein	carbs.	fiber
DAILY TOTALS					

Exercise and Fitness
DAILY PHYSICAL ACTIVITIES

ACTIVITY	cal. burned
TOTAL CAL. BURNED	

Vitamins/Supplements
DAILY INTAKE

DESCRIPTION	qty/time

ENERGY LEVELS ❑ low ❑ med ❑ high   WATER #OZ. _____

Daily Nutritional Intake

FOOD AND BEVERAGES   DATE   WEIGHT

MORNING/TIME:	cal.	fat	protein	carbs.	fiber
BREAKFAST TOTALS					

AFTERNOON/TIME:	cal.	fat	protein	carbs.	fiber
LUNCH TOTALS					

EVENING/TIME:	cal.	fat	protein	carbs.	fiber
DINNER TOTALS					

Daily Nutritional Intake
FOOD AND BEVERAGES

DAILY
GOALS
ACHIEVED

SNACKS/TIME:	cal.	fat	protein	carbs.	fiber
SNACK TOTALS					

	cal.	fat	protein	carbs.	fiber
DAILY TOTALS					

Exercise and Fitness
DAILY PHYSICAL ACTIVITIES

ACTIVITY	cal. burned
TOTAL CAL. BURNED	

Vitamins/Supplements
DAILY INTAKE

DESCRIPTION	qty/time

ENERGY LEVELS ❑ low ❑ med ❑ high   WATER #OZ. _____

Daily Nutritional Intake

FOOD AND BEVERAGES   DATE   WEIGHT

MORNING/TIME:	cal.	fat	protein	carbs.	fiber
BREAKFAST TOTALS					

AFTERNOON/TIME:	cal.	fat	protein	carbs.	fiber
LUNCH TOTALS					

EVENING/TIME:	cal.	fat	protein	carbs.	fiber
DINNER TOTALS					

Daily Nutritional Intake
FOOD AND BEVERAGES

DAILY
GOALS
ACHIEVED

SNACKS/TIME:	cal.	fat	protein	carbs.	fiber
SNACK TOTALS					

	cal.	fat	protein	carbs.	fiber
DAILY TOTALS					

Exercise and Fitness
DAILY PHYSICAL ACTIVITIES

ACTIVITY	cal. burned
TOTAL CAL. BURNED	

Vitamins/Supplements
DAILY INTAKE

DESCRIPTION	qty/time

ENERGY LEVELS ☐ low ☐ med ☐ high   WATER #OZ. _____

Daily Nutritional Intake

FOOD AND BEVERAGES   DATE   WEIGHT

MORNING/TIME:	cal.	fat	protein	carbs.	fiber
BREAKFAST TOTALS					

AFTERNOON/TIME:	cal.	fat	protein	carbs.	fiber
LUNCH TOTALS					

EVENING/TIME:	cal.	fat	protein	carbs.	fiber
DINNER TOTALS					

Daily Nutritional Intake
FOOD AND BEVERAGES

DAILY GOALS ACHIEVED I DID IT!

SNACKS/TIME:	cal.	fat	protein	carbs.	fiber
SNACK TOTALS					

	cal.	fat	protein	carbs.	fiber
DAILY TOTALS					

Exercise and Fitness
DAILY PHYSICAL ACTIVITIES

ACTIVITY	cal. burned
TOTAL CAL. BURNED	

Vitamins/Supplements
DAILY INTAKE

DESCRIPTION	qty/time

ENERGY LEVELS ❑ low ❑ med ❑ high   WATER #OZ. _____

Daily Nutritional Intake

FOOD AND BEVERAGES   DATE   WEIGHT

MORNING/TIME:	cal.	fat	protein	carbs.	fiber
BREAKFAST TOTALS					

AFTERNOON/TIME:	cal.	fat	protein	carbs.	fiber
LUNCH TOTALS					

EVENING/TIME:	cal.	fat	protein	carbs.	fiber
DINNER TOTALS					

Daily Nutritional Intake
FOOD AND BEVERAGES

SNACKS/TIME:	cal.	fat	protein	carbs.	fiber
SNACK TOTALS					

	cal.	fat	protein	carbs.	fiber
DAILY TOTALS					

Exercise and Fitness
DAILY PHYSICAL ACTIVITIES

ACTIVITY	cal. burned
TOTAL CAL. BURNED	

Vitamins/Supplements
DAILY INTAKE

DESCRIPTION	qty/time

ENERGY LEVELS ❑ low ❑ med ❑ high   WATER #OZ. _____

147

Daily Nutritional Intake

FOOD AND BEVERAGES

DATE   WEIGHT

MORNING/TIME:	cal.	fat	protein	carbs.	fiber
BREAKFAST TOTALS					

AFTERNOON/TIME:	cal.	fat	protein	carbs.	fiber
LUNCH TOTALS					

EVENING/TIME:	cal.	fat	protein	carbs.	fiber
DINNER TOTALS					

Daily Nutritional Intake
FOOD AND BEVERAGES

DAILY
GOALS
ACHIEVED

SNACKS/TIME:	cal.	fat	protein	carbs.	fiber
SNACK TOTALS					

	cal.	fat	protein	carbs.	fiber
DAILY TOTALS					

Exercise and Fitness
DAILY PHYSICAL ACTIVITIES

ACTIVITY	cal. burned
TOTAL CAL. BURNED	

Vitamins/Supplements
DAILY INTAKE

DESCRIPTION	qty/time

ENERGY LEVELS ❑ low ❑ med ❑ high   WATER #OZ. _____

Daily Nutritional Intake

FOOD AND BEVERAGES   DATE   WEIGHT

MORNING/TIME:	cal.	fat	protein	carbs.	fiber
BREAKFAST TOTALS					

AFTERNOON/TIME:	cal.	fat	protein	carbs.	fiber
LUNCH TOTALS					

EVENING/TIME:	cal.	fat	protein	carbs.	fiber
DINNER TOTALS					

Daily Nutritional Intake
FOOD AND BEVERAGES

DAILY
GOALS
ACHIEVED

SNACKS/TIME:	cal.	fat	protein	carbs.	fiber
SNACK TOTALS					

	cal.	fat	protein	carbs.	fiber
DAILY TOTALS					

Exercise and Fitness
DAILY PHYSICAL ACTIVITIES

ACTIVITY	cal. burned
TOTAL CAL. BURNED	

Vitamins/Supplements
DAILY INTAKE

DESCRIPTION	qty/time

ENERGY LEVELS ❑ low ❑ med ❑ high   WATER #OZ. _____

Daily Nutritional Intake

FOOD AND BEVERAGES   DATE   WEIGHT

MORNING/TIME:	cal.	fat	protein	carbs.	fiber
BREAKFAST TOTALS					

AFTERNOON/TIME:	cal.	fat	protein	carbs.	fiber
LUNCH TOTALS					

EVENING/TIME:	cal.	fat	protein	carbs.	fiber
DINNER TOTALS					

Daily Nutritional Intake
FOOD AND BEVERAGES

SNACKS/TIME:	cal.	fat	protein	carbs.	fiber
SNACK TOTALS					

	cal.	fat	protein	carbs.	fiber
DAILY TOTALS					

Exercise and Fitness
DAILY PHYSICAL ACTIVITIES

ACTIVITY	cal. burned
TOTAL CAL. BURNED	

Vitamins/Supplements
DAILY INTAKE

DESCRIPTION	qty/time

ENERGY LEVELS ❑ low ❑ med ❑ high   WATER #OZ. _____

153

Daily Nutritional Intake

FOOD AND BEVERAGES   DATE   WEIGHT

MORNING/TIME:	cal.	fat	protein	carbs.	fiber
BREAKFAST TOTALS					

AFTERNOON/TIME:	cal.	fat	protein	carbs.	fiber
LUNCH TOTALS					

EVENING/TIME:	cal.	fat	protein	carbs.	fiber
DINNER TOTALS					

Daily Nutritional Intake
FOOD AND BEVERAGES

DAILY
GOALS
ACHIEVED

SNACKS/TIME:	cal.	fat	protein	carbs.	fiber
SNACK TOTALS					

	cal.	fat	protein	carbs.	fiber
DAILY TOTALS					

Exercise and Fitness
DAILY PHYSICAL ACTIVITIES

ACTIVITY	cal. burned
TOTAL CAL. BURNED	

Vitamins/Supplements
DAILY INTAKE

DESCRIPTION	qty/time

ENERGY LEVELS ❑ low ❑ med ❑ high   WATER #OZ. _____

Daily Nutritional Intake

FOOD AND BEVERAGES

DATE   WEIGHT

MORNING/TIME:	cal.	fat	protein	carbs.	fiber
BREAKFAST TOTALS					

AFTERNOON/TIME:	cal.	fat	protein	carbs.	fiber
LUNCH TOTALS					

EVENING/TIME:	cal.	fat	protein	carbs.	fiber
DINNER TOTALS					

Daily Nutritional Intake
FOOD AND BEVERAGES

DAILY
GOALS
ACHIEVED

SNACKS/TIME:	cal.	fat	protein	carbs.	fiber
SNACK TOTALS					

	cal.	fat	protein	carbs.	fiber
DAILY TOTALS					

Exercise and Fitness
DAILY PHYSICAL ACTIVITIES

ACTIVITY	cal. burned
TOTAL CAL. BURNED	

Vitamins/Supplements
DAILY INTAKE

DESCRIPTION	qty/time

ENERGY LEVELS ❑ low ❑ med ❑ high   WATER #OZ. _____

157

Daily Nutritional Intake

FOOD AND BEVERAGES   DATE   WEIGHT

MORNING/TIME:	cal.	fat	protein	carbs.	fiber
BREAKFAST TOTALS					

AFTERNOON/TIME:	cal.	fat	protein	carbs.	fiber
LUNCH TOTALS					

EVENING/TIME:	cal.	fat	protein	carbs.	fiber
DINNER TOTALS					

Daily Nutritional Intake
FOOD AND BEVERAGES

DAILY GOALS ACHIEVED I DID IT!

SNACKS/TIME:	cal.	fat	protein	carbs.	fiber
SNACK TOTALS					

	cal.	fat	protein	carbs.	fiber
DAILY TOTALS					

Exercise and Fitness
DAILY PHYSICAL ACTIVITIES

ACTIVITY	cal. burned
TOTAL CAL. BURNED	

Vitamins/Supplements
DAILY INTAKE

DESCRIPTION	qty/time

ENERGY LEVELS ❑ low ❑ med ❑ high   WATER #OZ. _____

_____

_____

_____

_____

Daily Nutritional Intake

FOOD AND BEVERAGES   DATE   WEIGHT

MORNING/TIME:	cal.	fat	protein	carbs.	fiber
BREAKFAST TOTALS					

AFTERNOON/TIME:	cal.	fat	protein	carbs.	fiber
LUNCH TOTALS					

EVENING/TIME:	cal.	fat	protein	carbs.	fiber
DINNER TOTALS					

Daily Nutritional Intake
FOOD AND BEVERAGES

SNACKS/TIME:	cal.	fat	protein	carbs.	fiber
SNACK TOTALS					

	cal.	fat	protein	carbs.	fiber
DAILY TOTALS					

Exercise and Fitness
DAILY PHYSICAL ACTIVITIES

ACTIVITY	cal. burned
TOTAL CAL. BURNED	

Vitamins/Supplements
DAILY INTAKE

DESCRIPTION	qty/time

ENERGY LEVELS ❏ low ❏ med ❏ high   WATER #OZ. _____

Daily Nutritional Intake

FOOD AND BEVERAGES   DATE   WEIGHT

MORNING/TIME:	cal.	fat	protein	carbs.	fiber
BREAKFAST TOTALS					

AFTERNOON/TIME:	cal.	fat	protein	carbs.	fiber
LUNCH TOTALS					

EVENING/TIME:	cal.	fat	protein	carbs.	fiber
DINNER TOTALS					

Daily Nutritional Intake
FOOD AND BEVERAGES

DAILY
GOALS
ACHIEVED

SNACKS/TIME:	cal.	fat	protein	carbs.	fiber
SNACK TOTALS					

	cal.	fat	protein	carbs.	fiber
DAILY TOTALS					

Exercise and Fitness
DAILY PHYSICAL ACTIVITIES

ACTIVITY	cal. burned
TOTAL CAL. BURNED	

Vitamins/Supplements
DAILY INTAKE

DESCRIPTION	qty/time

ENERGY LEVELS ❑ low ❑ med ❑ high   WATER #OZ. _____

Daily Nutritional Intake

FOOD AND BEVERAGES

DATE   WEIGHT

MORNING/TIME:	cal.	fat	protein	carbs.	fiber
BREAKFAST TOTALS					

AFTERNOON/TIME:	cal.	fat	protein	carbs.	fiber
LUNCH TOTALS					

EVENING/TIME:	cal.	fat	protein	carbs.	fiber
DINNER TOTALS					

Daily Nutritional Intake
FOOD AND BEVERAGES

DAILY
GOALS
ACHIEVED

SNACKS/TIME:	cal.	fat	protein	carbs.	fiber
SNACK TOTALS					

	cal.	fat	protein	carbs.	fiber
DAILY TOTALS					

Exercise and Fitness
DAILY PHYSICAL ACTIVITIES

ACTIVITY	cal. burned
TOTAL CAL. BURNED	

Vitamins/Supplements
DAILY INTAKE

DESCRIPTION	qty/time

ENERGY LEVELS ❑ low ❑ med ❑ high   WATER #OZ. _____

165

Daily Nutritional Intake

FOOD AND BEVERAGES

DATE _____ WEIGHT _____

MORNING/TIME:	cal.	fat	protein	carbs.	fiber
BREAKFAST TOTALS					

AFTERNOON/TIME:	cal.	fat	protein	carbs.	fiber
LUNCH TOTALS					

EVENING/TIME:	cal.	fat	protein	carbs.	fiber
DINNER TOTALS					

Daily Nutritional Intake
FOOD AND BEVERAGES

SNACKS/TIME:	cal.	fat	protein	carbs.	fiber
SNACK TOTALS					

	cal.	fat	protein	carbs.	fiber
DAILY TOTALS					

Exercise and Fitness
DAILY PHYSICAL ACTIVITIES

ACTIVITY	cal. burned
TOTAL CAL. BURNED	

Vitamins/Supplements
DAILY INTAKE

DESCRIPTION	qty/time

ENERGY LEVELS ❑ low ❑ med ❑ high   WATER #OZ. _____

167

Daily Nutritional Intake

FOOD AND BEVERAGES

DATE   WEIGHT

MORNING/TIME:	cal.	fat	protein	carbs.	fiber
BREAKFAST TOTALS					

AFTERNOON/TIME:	cal.	fat	protein	carbs.	fiber
LUNCH TOTALS					

EVENING/TIME:	cal.	fat	protein	carbs.	fiber
DINNER TOTALS					

Daily Nutritional Intake
FOOD AND BEVERAGES

SNACKS/TIME:	cal.	fat	protein	carbs.	fiber
SNACK TOTALS					

	cal.	fat	protein	carbs.	fiber
DAILY TOTALS					

Exercise and Fitness
DAILY PHYSICAL ACTIVITIES

ACTIVITY	cal. burned
TOTAL CAL. BURNED	

Vitamins/Supplements
DAILY INTAKE

DESCRIPTION	qty/time

ENERGY LEVELS ❏ low ❏ med ❏ high   **WATER #OZ.** _____

Daily Nutritional Intake

FOOD AND BEVERAGES   DATE   WEIGHT

MORNING/TIME:	cal.	fat	protein	carbs.	fiber
BREAKFAST TOTALS					

AFTERNOON/TIME:	cal.	fat	protein	carbs.	fiber
LUNCH TOTALS					

EVENING/TIME:	cal.	fat	protein	carbs.	fiber
DINNER TOTALS					

Daily Nutritional Intake
FOOD AND BEVERAGES

DAILY
GOALS
ACHIEVED

SNACKS/TIME:	cal.	fat	protein	carbs.	fiber
SNACK TOTALS					

	cal.	fat	protein	carbs.	fiber
DAILY TOTALS					

Exercise and Fitness
DAILY PHYSICAL ACTIVITIES

ACTIVITY	cal. burned
TOTAL CAL. BURNED	

Vitamins/Supplements
DAILY INTAKE

DESCRIPTION	qty/time

ENERGY LEVELS ❑ low ❑ med ❑ high   WATER #OZ. _____

Daily Nutritional Intake

FOOD AND BEVERAGES

DATE _____ WEIGHT _____

MORNING/TIME:	cal.	fat	protein	carbs.	fiber
BREAKFAST TOTALS					

AFTERNOON/TIME:	cal.	fat	protein	carbs.	fiber
LUNCH TOTALS					

EVENING/TIME:	cal.	fat	protein	carbs.	fiber
DINNER TOTALS					

Daily Nutritional Intake
FOOD AND BEVERAGES

SNACKS/TIME:	cal.	fat	protein	carbs.	fiber
SNACK TOTALS					

	cal.	fat	protein	carbs.	fiber
DAILY TOTALS					

Exercise and Fitness
DAILY PHYSICAL ACTIVITIES

ACTIVITY	cal. burned
TOTAL CAL. BURNED	

Vitamins/Supplements
DAILY INTAKE

DESCRIPTION	qty/time

ENERGY LEVELS ❑ low ❑ med ❑ high   WATER #OZ. _____

173

Daily Nutritional Intake

FOOD AND BEVERAGES

DATE _____ WEIGHT

MORNING/TIME:	cal.	fat	protein	carbs.	fiber
BREAKFAST TOTALS					

AFTERNOON/TIME:	cal.	fat	protein	carbs.	fiber
LUNCH TOTALS					

EVENING/TIME:	cal.	fat	protein	carbs.	fiber
DINNER TOTALS					

Daily Nutritional Intake
FOOD AND BEVERAGES

SNACKS/TIME:	cal.	fat	protein	carbs.	fiber
SNACK TOTALS					

	cal.	fat	protein	carbs.	fiber
DAILY TOTALS					

Exercise and Fitness
DAILY PHYSICAL ACTIVITIES

ACTIVITY	cal. burned
TOTAL CAL. BURNED	

Vitamins/Supplements
DAILY INTAKE

DESCRIPTION	qty/time

ENERGY LEVELS ❏ low ❏ med ❏ high   WATER #OZ. _____

Daily Nutritional Intake

FOOD AND BEVERAGES   DATE   WEIGHT

MORNING/TIME:	cal.	fat	protein	carbs.	fiber
BREAKFAST TOTALS					

AFTERNOON/TIME:	cal.	fat	protein	carbs.	fiber
LUNCH TOTALS					

EVENING/TIME:	cal.	fat	protein	carbs.	fiber
DINNER TOTALS					

Daily Nutritional Intake
FOOD AND BEVERAGES

DAILY
GOALS
ACHIEVED

SNACKS/TIME:	cal.	fat	protein	carbs.	fiber
SNACK TOTALS					

	cal.	fat	protein	carbs.	fiber
DAILY TOTALS					

Exercise and Fitness
DAILY PHYSICAL ACTIVITIES

ACTIVITY	cal. burned
TOTAL CAL. BURNED	

Vitamins/Supplements
DAILY INTAKE

DESCRIPTION	qty/time

ENERGY LEVELS ❑ low ❑ med ❑ high   WATER #OZ. _____

177

Daily Nutritional Intake

FOOD AND BEVERAGES   DATE   WEIGHT

MORNING/TIME:	cal.	fat	protein	carbs.	fiber
BREAKFAST TOTALS					

AFTERNOON/TIME:	cal.	fat	protein	carbs.	fiber
LUNCH TOTALS					

EVENING/TIME:	cal.	fat	protein	carbs.	fiber
DINNER TOTALS					

Daily Nutritional Intake
FOOD AND BEVERAGES

DAILY
GOALS
ACHIEVED

 I DID IT!

SNACKS/TIME:	cal.	fat	protein	carbs.	fiber
SNACK TOTALS					

	cal.	fat	protein	carbs.	fiber
DAILY TOTALS					

Exercise and Fitness
DAILY PHYSICAL ACTIVITIES

ACTIVITY	cal. burned
TOTAL CAL. BURNED	

Vitamins/Supplements
DAILY INTAKE

DESCRIPTION	qty/time

ENERGY LEVELS ❏ low ❏ med ❏ high   WATER #OZ. _____

Daily Nutritional Intake
FOOD AND BEVERAGES

DATE   WEIGHT

MORNING/TIME:	cal.	fat	protein	carbs.	fiber
BREAKFAST TOTALS					

AFTERNOON/TIME:	cal.	fat	protein	carbs.	fiber
LUNCH TOTALS					

EVENING/TIME:	cal.	fat	protein	carbs.	fiber
DINNER TOTALS					

Daily Nutritional Intake
FOOD AND BEVERAGES

SNACKS/TIME:	cal.	fat	protein	carbs.	fiber
SNACK TOTALS					

	cal.	fat	protein	carbs.	fiber
DAILY TOTALS					

Exercise and Fitness
DAILY PHYSICAL ACTIVITIES

ACTIVITY	cal. burned
TOTAL CAL. BURNED	

Vitamins/Supplements
DAILY INTAKE

DESCRIPTION	qty/time

ENERGY LEVELS ❏ low ❏ med ❏ high   WATER #OZ. _____

181

Daily Nutritional Intake

FOOD AND BEVERAGES   DATE   WEIGHT

MORNING/TIME:	cal.	fat	protein	carbs.	fiber
BREAKFAST TOTALS					

AFTERNOON/TIME:	cal.	fat	protein	carbs.	fiber
LUNCH TOTALS					

EVENING/TIME:	cal.	fat	protein	carbs.	fiber
DINNER TOTALS					

Daily Nutritional Intake
FOOD AND BEVERAGES

DAILY
GOALS
ACHIEVED

SNACKS/TIME:	cal.	fat	protein	carbs.	fiber
SNACK TOTALS					

	cal.	fat	protein	carbs.	fiber
DAILY TOTALS					

Exercise and Fitness
DAILY PHYSICAL ACTIVITIES

ACTIVITY	cal. burned
TOTAL CAL. BURNED	

Vitamins/Supplements
DAILY INTAKE

DESCRIPTION	qty/time

ENERGY LEVELS ❑ low ❑ med ❑ high   WATER #OZ. _____

Daily Nutritional Intake

FOOD AND BEVERAGES   DATE   WEIGHT

MORNING/TIME:	cal.	fat	protein	carbs.	fiber
BREAKFAST TOTALS					

AFTERNOON/TIME:	cal.	fat	protein	carbs.	fiber
LUNCH TOTALS					

EVENING/TIME:	cal.	fat	protein	carbs.	fiber
DINNER TOTALS					

Daily Nutritional Intake
FOOD AND BEVERAGES

DAILY
GOALS
ACHIEVED

SNACKS/TIME:	cal.	fat	protein	carbs.	fiber
SNACK TOTALS					

	cal.	fat	protein	carbs.	fiber
DAILY TOTALS					

Exercise and Fitness
DAILY PHYSICAL ACTIVITIES

ACTIVITY	cal. burned
TOTAL CAL. BURNED	

Vitamins/Supplements
DAILY INTAKE

DESCRIPTION	qty/time

ENERGY LEVELS ❑ low ❑ med ❑ high   WATER #OZ. _____

Daily Nutritional Intake
FOOD AND BEVERAGES   DATE   WEIGHT

MORNING/TIME:	cal.	fat	protein	carbs.	fiber
BREAKFAST TOTALS					

AFTERNOON/TIME:	cal.	fat	protein	carbs.	fiber
LUNCH TOTALS					

EVENING/TIME:	cal.	fat	protein	carbs.	fiber
DINNER TOTALS					

Daily Nutritional Intake
FOOD AND BEVERAGES

SNACKS/TIME:	cal.	fat	protein	carbs.	fiber
SNACK TOTALS					

	cal.	fat	protein	carbs.	fiber
DAILY TOTALS					

Exercise and Fitness
DAILY PHYSICAL ACTIVITIES

ACTIVITY	cal. burned
TOTAL CAL. BURNED	

Vitamins/Supplements
DAILY INTAKE

DESCRIPTION	qty/time

ENERGY LEVELS ❑ low ❑ med ❑ high   WATER #OZ. _____

Daily Nutritional Intake

FOOD AND BEVERAGES   DATE   WEIGHT

MORNING/TIME:	cal.	fat	protein	carbs.	fiber
BREAKFAST TOTALS					

AFTERNOON/TIME:	cal.	fat	protein	carbs.	fiber
LUNCH TOTALS					

EVENING/TIME:	cal.	fat	protein	carbs.	fiber
DINNER TOTALS					

Daily Nutritional Intake
FOOD AND BEVERAGES

SNACKS/TIME:	cal.	fat	protein	carbs.	fiber
SNACK TOTALS					

	cal.	fat	protein	carbs.	fiber
DAILY TOTALS					

Exercise and Fitness
DAILY PHYSICAL ACTIVITIES

ACTIVITY	cal. burned
TOTAL CAL. BURNED	

Vitamins/Supplements
DAILY INTAKE

DESCRIPTION	qty/time

ENERGY LEVELS ❑ low ❑ med ❑ high   WATER #OZ. _____

189

Daily Nutritional Intake

FOOD AND BEVERAGES   DATE   WEIGHT

MORNING/TIME:	cal.	fat	protein	carbs.	fiber
BREAKFAST TOTALS					

AFTERNOON/TIME:	cal.	fat	protein	carbs.	fiber
LUNCH TOTALS					

EVENING/TIME:	cal.	fat	protein	carbs.	fiber
DINNER TOTALS					

Daily Nutritional Intake
FOOD AND BEVERAGES

SNACKS/TIME:	cal.	fat	protein	carbs.	fiber
SNACK TOTALS					

	cal.	fat	protein	carbs.	fiber
DAILY TOTALS					

Exercise and Fitness
DAILY PHYSICAL ACTIVITIES

ACTIVITY	cal. burned
TOTAL CAL. BURNED	

Vitamins/Supplements
DAILY INTAKE

DESCRIPTION	qty/time

ENERGY LEVELS ❑ low ❑ med ❑ high   WATER #OZ. _____

Daily Nutritional Intake

FOOD AND BEVERAGES   DATE   WEIGHT

MORNING/TIME:	cal.	fat	protein	carbs.	fiber
BREAKFAST TOTALS					

AFTERNOON/TIME:	cal.	fat	protein	carbs.	fiber
LUNCH TOTALS					

EVENING/TIME:	cal.	fat	protein	carbs.	fiber
DINNER TOTALS					

Daily Nutritional Intake
FOOD AND BEVERAGES

DAILY
GOALS
ACHIEVED

SNACKS/TIME:	cal.	fat	protein	carbs.	fiber
SNACK TOTALS					

	cal.	fat	protein	carbs.	fiber
DAILY TOTALS					

Exercise and Fitness
DAILY PHYSICAL ACTIVITIES

ACTIVITY	cal. burned
TOTAL CAL. BURNED	

Vitamins/Supplements
DAILY INTAKE

DESCRIPTION	qty/time

ENERGY LEVELS ❑ low ❑ med ❑ high   WATER #OZ. _____

193

Daily Nutritional Intake
FOOD AND BEVERAGES   DATE   WEIGHT

MORNING/TIME:	cal.	fat	protein	carbs.	fiber
BREAKFAST TOTALS					

AFTERNOON/TIME:	cal.	fat	protein	carbs.	fiber
LUNCH TOTALS					

EVENING/TIME:	cal.	fat	protein	carbs.	fiber
DINNER TOTALS					

Daily Nutritional Intake
FOOD AND BEVERAGES

SNACKS/TIME:	cal.	fat	protein	carbs.	fiber
SNACK TOTALS					

	cal.	fat	protein	carbs.	fiber
DAILY TOTALS					

Exercise and Fitness
DAILY PHYSICAL ACTIVITIES

ACTIVITY	cal. burned
TOTAL CAL. BURNED	

Vitamins/Supplements
DAILY INTAKE

DESCRIPTION	qty/time

ENERGY LEVELS ❑ low ❑ med ❑ high WATER #OZ. _____

Daily Nutritional Intake

FOOD AND BEVERAGES   DATE   WEIGHT

MORNING/TIME:	cal.	fat	protein	carbs.	fiber
BREAKFAST TOTALS					

AFTERNOON/TIME:	cal.	fat	protein	carbs.	fiber
LUNCH TOTALS					

EVENING/TIME:	cal.	fat	protein	carbs.	fiber
DINNER TOTALS					

Daily Nutritional Intake
FOOD AND BEVERAGES

SNACKS/TIME:	cal.	fat	protein	carbs.	fiber
SNACK TOTALS					

	cal.	fat	protein	carbs.	fiber
DAILY TOTALS					

Exercise and Fitness
DAILY PHYSICAL ACTIVITIES

ACTIVITY	cal. burned
TOTAL CAL. BURNED	

Vitamins/Supplements
DAILY INTAKE

DESCRIPTION	qty/time

ENERGY LEVELS ❑ low ❑ med ❑ high   **WATER #OZ.** _____

Daily Nutritional Intake

FOOD AND BEVERAGES

DATE _____ WEIGHT _____

MORNING/TIME:	cal.	fat	protein	carbs.	fiber
BREAKFAST TOTALS					

AFTERNOON/TIME:	cal.	fat	protein	carbs.	fiber
LUNCH TOTALS					

EVENING/TIME:	cal.	fat	protein	carbs.	fiber
DINNER TOTALS					

Daily Nutritional Intake
FOOD AND BEVERAGES

DAILY
GOALS
ACHIEVED

SNACKS/TIME:	cal.	fat	protein	carbs.	fiber
SNACK TOTALS					

	cal.	fat	protein	carbs.	fiber
DAILY TOTALS					

Exercise and Fitness
DAILY PHYSICAL ACTIVITIES

ACTIVITY	cal. burned
TOTAL CAL. BURNED	

Vitamins/Supplements
DAILY INTAKE

DESCRIPTION	qty/time

ENERGY LEVELS ❑ low ❑ med ❑ high   WATER #OZ. _____

Daily Nutritional Intake

FOOD AND BEVERAGES   DATE   WEIGHT

MORNING/TIME:	cal.	fat	protein	carbs.	fiber
BREAKFAST TOTALS					

AFTERNOON/TIME:	cal.	fat	protein	carbs.	fiber
LUNCH TOTALS					

EVENING/TIME:	cal.	fat	protein	carbs.	fiber
DINNER TOTALS					

Daily Nutritional Intake
FOOD AND BEVERAGES

DAILY
GOALS
ACHIEVED

SNACKS/TIME:	cal.	fat	protein	carbs.	fiber
SNACK TOTALS					

	cal.	fat	protein	carbs.	fiber
DAILY TOTALS					

Exercise and Fitness
DAILY PHYSICAL ACTIVITIES

ACTIVITY	cal. burned
TOTAL CAL. BURNED	

Vitamins/Supplements
DAILY INTAKE

DESCRIPTION	qty/time

ENERGY LEVELS ☐ low ☐ med ☐ high   WATER #OZ. _____

_____

_____

_____

_____

201

Daily Nutritional Intake
FOOD AND BEVERAGES   DATE   WEIGHT

MORNING/TIME:	cal.	fat	protein	carbs.	fiber
BREAKFAST TOTALS					

AFTERNOON/TIME:	cal.	fat	protein	carbs.	fiber
LUNCH TOTALS					

EVENING/TIME:	cal.	fat	protein	carbs.	fiber
DINNER TOTALS					

Daily Nutritional Intake
FOOD AND BEVERAGES

DAILY GOALS ACHIEVED

SNACKS/TIME:	cal.	fat	protein	carbs.	fiber
SNACK TOTALS					

	cal.	fat	protein	carbs.	fiber
DAILY TOTALS					

Exercise and Fitness
DAILY PHYSICAL ACTIVITIES

ACTIVITY	cal. burned
TOTAL CAL. BURNED	

Vitamins/Supplements
DAILY INTAKE

DESCRIPTION	qty/time

ENERGY LEVELS ❑ low ❑ med ❑ high   **WATER #OZ.** _____

Daily Nutritional Intake

FOOD AND BEVERAGES

DATE _____ WEIGHT _____

MORNING/TIME:	cal.	fat	protein	carbs.	fiber
BREAKFAST TOTALS					

AFTERNOON/TIME:	cal.	fat	protein	carbs.	fiber
LUNCH TOTALS					

EVENING/TIME:	cal.	fat	protein	carbs.	fiber
DINNER TOTALS					

Daily Nutritional Intake
FOOD AND BEVERAGES

DAILY
GOALS
ACHIEVED

I DID IT!

SNACKS/TIME:	cal.	fat	protein	carbs.	fiber
SNACK TOTALS					

	cal.	fat	protein	carbs.	fiber
DAILY TOTALS					

Exercise and Fitness
DAILY PHYSICAL ACTIVITIES

ACTIVITY	cal. burned
TOTAL CAL. BURNED	

Vitamins/Supplements
DAILY INTAKE

DESCRIPTION	qty/time

ENERGY LEVELS ❑ low ❑ med ❑ high   WATER #OZ. _____

205

Daily Nutritional Intake

FOOD AND BEVERAGES   DATE   WEIGHT

MORNING/TIME:	cal.	fat	protein	carbs.	fiber
BREAKFAST TOTALS					

AFTERNOON/TIME:	cal.	fat	protein	carbs.	fiber
LUNCH TOTALS					

EVENING/TIME:	cal.	fat	protein	carbs.	fiber
DINNER TOTALS					

Daily Nutritional Intake
FOOD AND BEVERAGES

DAILY
GOALS
ACHIEVED

SNACKS/TIME:	cal.	fat	protein	carbs.	fiber
SNACK TOTALS					

	cal.	fat	protein	carbs.	fiber
DAILY TOTALS					

Exercise and Fitness
DAILY PHYSICAL ACTIVITIES

ACTIVITY	cal. burned
TOTAL CAL. BURNED	

Vitamins/Supplements
DAILY INTAKE

DESCRIPTION	qty/time

ENERGY LEVELS ☐ low ☐ med ☐ high   WATER #OZ. _____

_____

_____

_____

_____

Daily Nutritional Intake

FOOD AND BEVERAGES

DATE _____   WEIGHT _____

MORNING/TIME:	cal.	fat	protein	carbs.	fiber
BREAKFAST TOTALS					

AFTERNOON/TIME:	cal.	fat	protein	carbs.	fiber
LUNCH TOTALS					

EVENING/TIME:	cal.	fat	protein	carbs.	fiber
DINNER TOTALS					

Daily Nutritional Intake
FOOD AND BEVERAGES

SNACKS/TIME:	cal.	fat	protein	carbs.	fiber
SNACK TOTALS					

	cal.	fat	protein	carbs.	fiber
DAILY TOTALS					

Exercise and Fitness
DAILY PHYSICAL ACTIVITIES

ACTIVITY	cal. burned
TOTAL CAL. BURNED	

Vitamins/Supplements
DAILY INTAKE

DESCRIPTION	qty/time

ENERGY LEVELS ❑ low ❑ med ❑ high **WATER #OZ.** _____

Daily Nutritional Intake
FOOD AND BEVERAGES

DATE _____ WEIGHT _____

MORNING/TIME:	cal.	fat	protein	carbs.	fiber
BREAKFAST TOTALS					

AFTERNOON/TIME:	cal.	fat	protein	carbs.	fiber
LUNCH TOTALS					

EVENING/TIME:	cal.	fat	protein	carbs.	fiber
DINNER TOTALS					

Daily Nutritional Intake
FOOD AND BEVERAGES

DAILY GOALS ACHIEVED

SNACKS/TIME:	cal.	fat	protein	carbs.	fiber
SNACK TOTALS					

	cal.	fat	protein	carbs.	fiber
DAILY TOTALS					

Exercise and Fitness
DAILY PHYSICAL ACTIVITIES

ACTIVITY	cal. burned
TOTAL CAL. BURNED	

Vitamins/Supplements
DAILY INTAKE

DESCRIPTION	qty/time

ENERGY LEVELS ❑ low ❑ med ❑ high   WATER #OZ. _____

_____

_____

_____

_____

211

Daily Nutritional Intake

FOOD AND BEVERAGES   DATE   WEIGHT

MORNING/TIME:	cal.	fat	protein	carbs.	fiber
BREAKFAST TOTALS					

AFTERNOON/TIME:	cal.	fat	protein	carbs.	fiber
LUNCH TOTALS					

EVENING/TIME:	cal.	fat	protein	carbs.	fiber
DINNER TOTALS					

Daily Nutritional Intake
FOOD AND BEVERAGES

SNACKS/TIME:	cal.	fat	protein	carbs.	fiber
SNACK TOTALS					

	cal.	fat	protein	carbs.	fiber
DAILY TOTALS					

Exercise and Fitness
DAILY PHYSICAL ACTIVITIES

ACTIVITY	cal. burned
TOTAL CAL. BURNED	

Vitamins/Supplements
DAILY INTAKE

DESCRIPTION	qty/time

ENERGY LEVELS ❑ low ❑ med ❑ high   WATER #OZ. _____

Daily Nutritional Intake

FOOD AND BEVERAGES

DATE   WEIGHT

MORNING/TIME:	cal.	fat	protein	carbs.	fiber
BREAKFAST TOTALS					

AFTERNOON/TIME:	cal.	fat	protein	carbs.	fiber
LUNCH TOTALS					

EVENING/TIME:	cal.	fat	protein	carbs.	fiber
DINNER TOTALS					

Daily Nutritional Intake
FOOD AND BEVERAGES

SNACKS/TIME:	cal.	fat	protein	carbs.	fiber
SNACK TOTALS					

	cal.	fat	protein	carbs.	fiber
DAILY TOTALS					

Exercise and Fitness
DAILY PHYSICAL ACTIVITIES

ACTIVITY	cal. burned
TOTAL CAL. BURNED	

Vitamins/Supplements
DAILY INTAKE

DESCRIPTION	qty/time

ENERGY LEVELS ❏ low ❏ med ❏ high   WATER #OZ. _____

215

Daily Nutritional Intake
FOOD AND BEVERAGES   DATE   WEIGHT

MORNING/TIME:	cal.	fat	protein	carbs.	fiber
BREAKFAST TOTALS					

AFTERNOON/TIME:	cal.	fat	protein	carbs.	fiber
LUNCH TOTALS					

EVENING/TIME:	cal.	fat	protein	carbs.	fiber
DINNER TOTALS					

Daily Nutritional Intake
FOOD AND BEVERAGES

DAILY
GOALS
ACHIEVED

SNACKS/TIME:	cal.	fat	protein	carbs.	fiber
SNACK TOTALS					

	cal.	fat	protein	carbs.	fiber
DAILY TOTALS					

Exercise and Fitness
DAILY PHYSICAL ACTIVITIES

ACTIVITY	cal. burned
TOTAL CAL. BURNED	

Vitamins/Supplements
DAILY INTAKE

DESCRIPTION	qty/time

ENERGY LEVELS ☐ low ☐ med ☐ high   WATER #OZ. _____

217

Daily Nutritional Intake
FOOD AND BEVERAGES   DATE   WEIGHT

MORNING/TIME:	cal.	fat	protein	carbs.	fiber
BREAKFAST TOTALS					

AFTERNOON/TIME:	cal.	fat	protein	carbs.	fiber
LUNCH TOTALS					

EVENING/TIME:	cal.	fat	protein	carbs.	fiber
DINNER TOTALS					

Daily Nutritional Intake
FOOD AND BEVERAGES

SNACKS/TIME:	cal.	fat	protein	carbs.	fiber
SNACK TOTALS					

	cal.	fat	protein	carbs.	fiber
DAILY TOTALS					

Exercise and Fitness
DAILY PHYSICAL ACTIVITIES

ACTIVITY	cal. burned
TOTAL CAL. BURNED	

Vitamins/Supplements
DAILY INTAKE

DESCRIPTION	qty/time

ENERGY LEVELS ❑ low ❑ med ❑ high   **WATER #OZ.** _____

Daily Nutritional Intake

FOOD AND BEVERAGES

DATE　　　WEIGHT

MORNING/TIME:	cal.	fat	protein	carbs.	fiber
BREAKFAST TOTALS					

AFTERNOON/TIME:	cal.	fat	protein	carbs.	fiber
LUNCH TOTALS					

EVENING/TIME:	cal.	fat	protein	carbs.	fiber
DINNER TOTALS					

Daily Nutritional Intake
FOOD AND BEVERAGES

SNACKS/TIME:	cal.	fat	protein	carbs.	fiber
SNACK TOTALS					

	cal.	fat	protein	carbs.	fiber
DAILY TOTALS					

Exercise and Fitness
DAILY PHYSICAL ACTIVITIES

ACTIVITY	cal. burned
TOTAL CAL. BURNED	

Vitamins/Supplements
DAILY INTAKE

DESCRIPTION	qty/time

ENERGY LEVELS ❑ low ❑ med ❑ high   WATER #OZ. _____

221

Daily Nutritional Intake

FOOD AND BEVERAGES

DATE _____ WEIGHT _____

MORNING/TIME:	cal.	fat	protein	carbs.	fiber
BREAKFAST TOTALS					

AFTERNOON/TIME:	cal.	fat	protein	carbs.	fiber
LUNCH TOTALS					

EVENING/TIME:	cal.	fat	protein	carbs.	fiber
DINNER TOTALS					

Daily Nutritional Intake
FOOD AND BEVERAGES

SNACKS/TIME:	cal.	fat	protein	carbs.	fiber
SNACK TOTALS					

	cal.	fat	protein	carbs.	fiber
DAILY TOTALS					

Exercise and Fitness
DAILY PHYSICAL ACTIVITIES

ACTIVITY	cal. burned
TOTAL CAL. BURNED	

Vitamins/Supplements
DAILY INTAKE

DESCRIPTION	qty/time

ENERGY LEVELS ☐ low ☐ med ☐ high   **WATER #OZ.** _____

Daily Nutritional Intake

FOOD AND BEVERAGES   DATE   WEIGHT

MORNING/TIME:	cal.	fat	protein	carbs.	fiber
BREAKFAST TOTALS					

AFTERNOON/TIME:	cal.	fat	protein	carbs.	fiber
LUNCH TOTALS					

EVENING/TIME:	cal.	fat	protein	carbs.	fiber
DINNER TOTALS					

Daily Nutritional Intake
FOOD AND BEVERAGES

SNACKS/TIME:	cal.	fat	protein	carbs.	fiber
SNACK TOTALS					

	cal.	fat	protein	carbs.	fiber
DAILY TOTALS					

Exercise and Fitness
DAILY PHYSICAL ACTIVITIES

ACTIVITY	cal. burned
TOTAL CAL. BURNED	

Vitamins/Supplements
DAILY INTAKE

DESCRIPTION	qty/time

ENERGY LEVELS ☐ low ☐ med ☐ high   WATER #OZ. _____

Daily Nutritional Intake

FOOD AND BEVERAGES   DATE   WEIGHT

MORNING/TIME:	cal.	fat	protein	carbs.	fiber
BREAKFAST TOTALS					

AFTERNOON/TIME:	cal.	fat	protein	carbs.	fiber
LUNCH TOTALS					

EVENING/TIME:	cal.	fat	protein	carbs.	fiber
DINNER TOTALS					

Daily Nutritional Intake
FOOD AND BEVERAGES

SNACKS/TIME:	cal.	fat	protein	carbs.	fiber
SNACK TOTALS					

	cal.	fat	protein	carbs.	fiber
DAILY TOTALS					

Exercise and Fitness
DAILY PHYSICAL ACTIVITIES

ACTIVITY	cal. burned
TOTAL CAL. BURNED	

Vitamins/Supplements
DAILY INTAKE

DESCRIPTION	qty/time

ENERGY LEVELS ❑ low ❑ med ❑ high   WATER #OZ. _____

227

Daily Nutritional Intake

FOOD AND BEVERAGES   DATE   WEIGHT

MORNING/TIME:	cal.	fat	protein	carbs.	fiber
BREAKFAST TOTALS					

AFTERNOON/TIME:	cal.	fat	protein	carbs.	fiber
LUNCH TOTALS					

EVENING/TIME:	cal.	fat	protein	carbs.	fiber
DINNER TOTALS					

Daily Nutritional Intake
FOOD AND BEVERAGES

DAILY GOALS ACHIEVED

SNACKS/TIME:	cal.	fat	protein	carbs.	fiber
SNACK TOTALS					

	cal.	fat	protein	carbs.	fiber
DAILY TOTALS					

Exercise and Fitness
DAILY PHYSICAL ACTIVITIES

ACTIVITY	cal. burned
TOTAL CAL. BURNED	

Vitamins/Supplements
DAILY INTAKE

DESCRIPTION	qty/time

ENERGY LEVELS ☐ low ☐ med ☐ high   WATER #OZ. _____

Daily Nutritional Intake

FOOD AND BEVERAGES   DATE   WEIGHT

MORNING/TIME:	cal.	fat	protein	carbs.	fiber
BREAKFAST TOTALS					

AFTERNOON/TIME:	cal.	fat	protein	carbs.	fiber
LUNCH TOTALS					

EVENING/TIME:	cal.	fat	protein	carbs.	fiber
DINNER TOTALS					

Daily Nutritional Intake
FOOD AND BEVERAGES

DAILY
GOALS
ACHIEVED

SNACKS/TIME:	cal.	fat	protein	carbs.	fiber
SNACK TOTALS					

	cal.	fat	protein	carbs.	fiber
DAILY TOTALS					

Exercise and Fitness
DAILY PHYSICAL ACTIVITIES

ACTIVITY	cal. burned
TOTAL CAL. BURNED	

Vitamins/Supplements
DAILY INTAKE

DESCRIPTION	qty/time

ENERGY LEVELS ❑ low ❑ med ❑ high   WATER #OZ. _____

231

Daily Nutritional Intake

FOOD AND BEVERAGES DATE   WEIGHT

MORNING/TIME:	cal.	fat	protein	carbs.	fiber
BREAKFAST TOTALS					

AFTERNOON/TIME:	cal.	fat	protein	carbs.	fiber
LUNCH TOTALS					

EVENING/TIME:	cal.	fat	protein	carbs.	fiber
DINNER TOTALS					

Daily Nutritional Intake
FOOD AND BEVERAGES

SNACKS/TIME:	cal.	fat	protein	carbs.	fiber
SNACK TOTALS					

	cal.	fat	protein	carbs.	fiber
DAILY TOTALS					

Exercise and Fitness
DAILY PHYSICAL ACTIVITIES

ACTIVITY	cal. burned
TOTAL CAL. BURNED	

Vitamins/Supplements
DAILY INTAKE

DESCRIPTION	qty/time

ENERGY LEVELS ❑ low ❑ med ❑ high   WATER #OZ. _____

Daily Nutritional Intake

FOOD AND BEVERAGES

DATE   WEIGHT

MORNING/TIME:	cal.	fat	protein	carbs.	fiber
BREAKFAST TOTALS					

AFTERNOON/TIME:	cal.	fat	protein	carbs.	fiber
LUNCH TOTALS					

EVENING/TIME:	cal.	fat	protein	carbs.	fiber
DINNER TOTALS					

Daily Nutritional Intake
FOOD AND BEVERAGES

DAILY
GOALS
ACHIEVED

SNACKS/TIME:	cal.	fat	protein	carbs.	fiber
SNACK TOTALS					

	cal.	fat	protein	carbs.	fiber
DAILY TOTALS					

Exercise and Fitness
DAILY PHYSICAL ACTIVITIES

ACTIVITY	cal. burned
TOTAL CAL. BURNED	

Vitamins/Supplements
DAILY INTAKE

DESCRIPTION	qty/time

ENERGY LEVELS ❏ low ❏ med ❏ high   WATER #OZ. _____

Daily Nutritional Intake

FOOD AND BEVERAGES

DATE _____ WEIGHT _____

MORNING/TIME:	cal.	fat	protein	carbs.	fiber
BREAKFAST TOTALS					

AFTERNOON/TIME:	cal.	fat	protein	carbs.	fiber
LUNCH TOTALS					

EVENING/TIME:	cal.	fat	protein	carbs.	fiber
DINNER TOTALS					

Daily Nutritional Intake
FOOD AND BEVERAGES

SNACKS/TIME:	cal.	fat	protein	carbs.	fiber
SNACK TOTALS					

	cal.	fat	protein	carbs.	fiber
DAILY TOTALS					

Exercise and Fitness
DAILY PHYSICAL ACTIVITIES

ACTIVITY	cal. burned
TOTAL CAL. BURNED	

Vitamins/Supplements
DAILY INTAKE

DESCRIPTION	qty/time

ENERGY LEVELS ❑ low ❑ med ❑ high   WATER #OZ. _____

Daily Nutritional Intake

FOOD AND BEVERAGES

DATE   WEIGHT

MORNING/TIME:	cal.	fat	protein	carbs.	fiber
BREAKFAST TOTALS					

AFTERNOON/TIME:	cal.	fat	protein	carbs.	fiber
LUNCH TOTALS					

EVENING/TIME:	cal.	fat	protein	carbs.	fiber
DINNER TOTALS					

Daily Nutritional Intake
FOOD AND BEVERAGES

SNACKS/TIME:	cal.	fat	protein	carbs.	fiber
SNACK TOTALS					

	cal.	fat	protein	carbs.	fiber
DAILY TOTALS					

Exercise and Fitness
DAILY PHYSICAL ACTIVITIES

ACTIVITY	cal. burned
TOTAL CAL. BURNED	

Vitamins/Supplements
DAILY INTAKE

DESCRIPTION	qty/time

ENERGY LEVELS ❑ low ❑ med ❑ high WATER #OZ. _____

239

Daily Nutritional Intake

FOOD AND BEVERAGES   DATE   WEIGHT

MORNING/TIME:	cal.	fat	protein	carbs.	fiber
BREAKFAST TOTALS					

AFTERNOON/TIME:	cal.	fat	protein	carbs.	fiber
LUNCH TOTALS					

EVENING/TIME:	cal.	fat	protein	carbs.	fiber
DINNER TOTALS					

Daily Nutritional Intake
FOOD AND BEVERAGES

SNACKS/TIME:	cal.	fat	protein	carbs.	fiber
SNACK TOTALS					

	cal.	fat	protein	carbs.	fiber
DAILY TOTALS					

Exercise and Fitness
DAILY PHYSICAL ACTIVITIES

ACTIVITY	cal. burned
TOTAL CAL. BURNED	

Vitamins/Supplements
DAILY INTAKE

DESCRIPTION	qty/time

ENERGY LEVELS ❑ low ❑ med ❑ high   WATER #OZ. _____

241

Daily Nutritional Intake

FOOD AND BEVERAGES DATE WEIGHT

MORNING/TIME:	cal.	fat	protein	carbs.	fiber
BREAKFAST TOTALS					

AFTERNOON/TIME:	cal.	fat	protein	carbs.	fiber
					.
LUNCH TOTALS					

EVENING/TIME:	cal.	fat	protein	carbs.	fiber
DINNER TOTALS					

Daily Nutritional Intake
FOOD AND BEVERAGES

SNACKS/TIME:	cal.	fat	protein	carbs.	fiber
SNACK TOTALS					

	cal.	fat	protein	carbs.	fiber
DAILY TOTALS					

Exercise and Fitness
DAILY PHYSICAL ACTIVITIES

ACTIVITY	cal. burned
TOTAL CAL. BURNED	

Vitamins/Supplements
DAILY INTAKE

DESCRIPTION	qty/time

ENERGY LEVELS ☐ low ☐ med ☐ high   WATER #OZ. _____

Daily Nutritional Intake
FOOD AND BEVERAGES   DATE   WEIGHT

MORNING/TIME:	cal.	fat	protein	carbs.	fiber
BREAKFAST TOTALS					

AFTERNOON/TIME:	cal.	fat	protein	carbs.	fiber
LUNCH TOTALS					

EVENING/TIME:	cal.	fat	protein	carbs.	fiber
DINNER TOTALS					

Daily Nutritional Intake
FOOD AND BEVERAGES

DAILY
GOALS
ACHIEVED

SNACKS/TIME:	cal.	fat	protein	carbs.	fiber
SNACK TOTALS					

	cal.	fat	protein	carbs.	fiber
DAILY TOTALS					

Exercise and Fitness
DAILY PHYSICAL ACTIVITIES

ACTIVITY	cal. burned
TOTAL CAL. BURNED	

Vitamins/Supplements
DAILY INTAKE

DESCRIPTION	qty/time

ENERGY LEVELS ❑ low ❑ med ❑ high   WATER #OZ. _____

Daily Nutritional Intake

FOOD AND BEVERAGES

DATE   WEIGHT

MORNING/TIME:	cal.	fat	protein	carbs.	fiber
BREAKFAST TOTALS					

AFTERNOON/TIME:	cal.	fat	protein	carbs.	fiber
LUNCH TOTALS					

EVENING/TIME:	cal.	fat	protein	carbs.	fiber
DINNER TOTALS					

Daily Nutritional Intake
FOOD AND BEVERAGES

SNACKS/TIME:	cal.	fat	protein	carbs.	fiber
SNACK TOTALS					

	cal.	fat	protein	carbs.	fiber
DAILY TOTALS					

Exercise and Fitness
DAILY PHYSICAL ACTIVITIES

ACTIVITY	cal. burned
TOTAL CAL. BURNED	

Vitamins/Supplements
DAILY INTAKE

DESCRIPTION	qty/time

ENERGY LEVELS ☐ low ☐ med ☐ high   WATER #OZ. _____

247

Daily Nutritional Intake

FOOD AND BEVERAGES   DATE   WEIGHT

MORNING/TIME:	cal.	fat	protein	carbs.	fiber
BREAKFAST TOTALS					

AFTERNOON/TIME:	cal.	fat	protein	carbs.	fiber
LUNCH TOTALS					

EVENING/TIME:	cal.	fat	protein	carbs.	fiber
DINNER TOTALS					

Daily Nutritional Intake
FOOD AND BEVERAGES

DAILY
GOALS
ACHIEVED

SNACKS/TIME:	cal.	fat	protein	carbs.	fiber
SNACK TOTALS					

	cal.	fat	protein	carbs.	fiber
DAILY TOTALS					

Exercise and Fitness
DAILY PHYSICAL ACTIVITIES

ACTIVITY	cal. burned
TOTAL CAL. BURNED	

Vitamins/Supplements
DAILY INTAKE

DESCRIPTION	qty/time

ENERGY LEVELS ❑ low ❑ med ❑ high   WATER #OZ. _____

Daily Nutritional Intake

FOOD AND BEVERAGES

DATE   WEIGHT

MORNING/TIME:	cal.	fat	protein	carbs.	fiber
BREAKFAST TOTALS					

AFTERNOON/TIME:	cal.	fat	protein	carbs.	fiber
LUNCH TOTALS					

EVENING/TIME:	cal.	fat	protein	carbs.	fiber
DINNER TOTALS					

Daily Nutritional Intake
FOOD AND BEVERAGES

SNACKS/TIME:	cal.	fat	protein	carbs.	fiber
SNACK TOTALS					

	cal.	fat	protein	carbs.	fiber
DAILY TOTALS					

Exercise and Fitness
DAILY PHYSICAL ACTIVITIES

ACTIVITY	cal. burned
TOTAL CAL. BURNED	

Vitamins/Supplements
DAILY INTAKE

DESCRIPTION	qty/time

ENERGY LEVELS ❑ low ❑ med ❑ high   WATER #OZ. _____

Daily Nutritional Intake

FOOD AND BEVERAGES

DATE   WEIGHT

MORNING/TIME:	cal.	fat	protein	carbs.	fiber
BREAKFAST TOTALS					

AFTERNOON/TIME:	cal.	fat	protein	carbs.	fiber
LUNCH TOTALS					

EVENING/TIME:	cal.	fat	protein	carbs.	fiber
DINNER TOTALS					

Daily Nutritional Intake
FOOD AND BEVERAGES

SNACKS/TIME:	cal.	fat	protein	carbs.	fiber
SNACK TOTALS					

	cal.	fat	protein	carbs.	fiber
DAILY TOTALS					

Exercise and Fitness
DAILY PHYSICAL ACTIVITIES

Vitamins/Supplements
DAILY INTAKE

ACTIVITY	cal. burned
TOTAL CAL. BURNED	

DESCRIPTION	qty/time

ENERGY LEVELS ❑ low ❑ med ❑ high   WATER #OZ. _____

_____

_____

_____

_____

Daily Nutritional Intake

FOOD AND BEVERAGES   DATE   WEIGHT

MORNING/TIME:	cal.	fat	protein	carbs.	fiber
BREAKFAST TOTALS					

AFTERNOON/TIME:	cal.	fat	protein	carbs.	fiber
LUNCH TOTALS					

EVENING/TIME:	cal.	fat	protein	carbs.	fiber
DINNER TOTALS					

Daily Nutritional Intake
FOOD AND BEVERAGES

SNACKS/TIME:	cal.	fat	protein	carbs.	fiber
SNACK TOTALS					

	cal.	fat	protein	carbs.	fiber
DAILY TOTALS					

Exercise and Fitness
DAILY PHYSICAL ACTIVITIES

ACTIVITY	cal. burned
TOTAL CAL. BURNED	

Vitamins/Supplements
DAILY INTAKE

DESCRIPTION	qty/time

ENERGY LEVELS ❑ low ❑ med ❑ high   WATER #OZ. _____

255

NUTRITIONAL FACTS ON

POPULAR FOOD ITEMS

This section is a great resource for nutritional information on foods you may want to select for your weight-loss program. It will provide calories per serving, as well as the content in grams for protein, fats, carbohydrates, and fiber.

To use this section, look up food items which are listed in alphabetical order. Locate the corresponding information, and log the data into your journal so you can track your daily totals.

Nutrition values for fat, protein, carbohydrates, and fiber are listed in grams per serving. Serving sizes and values are approximate.

FOOD ITEM	Serving Size	Cal.	Fat	Protein	Carbs	Fiber
A						
Alcohol, 100 proof	1 fl oz	82	0	0	0	0
Alcohol, 86 proof	1 fl oz	70	0	0	0	0
Alcohol, 90 proof	1 fl oz	73	0	0	0	0
Alcohol, 94 proof	1 fl oz	76	0	0	0	0
Alcohol, dessert wine, dry	1 glass	157	0	0.2	12	0
Alcohol, dessert wine, sweet	1 glass	165	0	0.2	14.1	0
Alcohol, liquors	1 fl oz	107	0.1	0	11.2	0
Alcohol, pina colada	8 fl oz	440	4.8	1	57	0.4
Alfalfa seeds	1 tbsp	1	0	0.1	0.1	0.1
Allspice, ground	1 tsp	5	0.2	0.1	1.4	0.4
Almond butter, w/ salt	1 tbsp	101	9.5	2.4	3.4	0.6
Almond butter, w/o salt	1 tbsp	101	9.5	2.4	3.4	0.6
Almonds, roasted	1 oz (12 nuts)	169	15	6.2	5.5	3.3
Anchovies	3 oz	111	4.1	17.3	0	0
Apple cider, powdered	1 packet	83	0	0	20.7	0
Apple juice	8 fl oz	120	0.2	0.2	28.8	0
Apples, w/o skin	1 medium	61	0.2	0.3	16	1.7
Apples, w/ skin	1 medium	72	0.2	0.4	19	3.3
Applesauce	1 cup	194	0.5	0.5	50.8	3.1
Apricots	1 apricot	17	0.1	0.5	3.9	0.7
Arrowroot	1 cup, sliced	78	0.2	5.1	16.1	1.6
Arrowroot flour	1 cup	457	0.1	0.4	112.8	4.4
Artichokes	1 artichoke	76	0.2	5.3	17	8.7
Arugula	1 cup	4	0.1	0.5	0.7	0.4
Asparagus	1 spear	2	0	0.3	0.5	0.3
Avocados	1 cup, cubes	240	22	3	12.8	10
B						
Bacon bits, meatless	1 tbsp	33	1.8	2.2	2	0.7
Bacon, canadian, cooked	1 slice	43	2	5.8	0.3	0
Bacon, meatless	1 slice	16	1.5	0.5	0.3	0.1
Bacon, pork, cooked	1 slice	42	3.2	3	0.1	0
Bagels, cinnamon-raisin	1 bagel, 4" dia	244	1.5	8.7	49	2
Bagels, egg	1 bagel, 4" dia	292	2.2	11	55.6	2.4
Bagels, oat-bran	1 bagel, 4" dia	227	1	9.5	47	3.2
Bagels, plain	1 bagel, 4" dia	245	1.4	9.3	47	2
Bagels, deli gourmet style	1 bagel	370	3	13	71	2
Balsam-pear	1 balsam-pear	21	0.2	1.2	4.6	3.5
Bamboo shoots	1 cup	41	0.5	3.9	7.9	3.3
Banana chips	1 oz	147	9.5	0.7	16.6	2.2
Bananas	1 medium, 7"-8"	105	0.4	13	27	3
Barley	1 cup	651	4.2	23	135.2	31.8
Barley flour	1 cup	511	2.4	15.5	110.3	14.9
Barley, pearled, cooked	1 cup	193	0.7	3.6	44.3	6
Basil	5 leaves	1	0	0.1	0.1	0.1
Basil, dried	1 tsp	2	0	0.1	0.4	0.3
Bay leaf	1 tsp, crumbled	2	0.1	0	0.4	0.2
Beans, adzuki, cooked	1 cup	294	0.2	17	57	16.8
Beans, baked, canned, plain	1 cup	239	0.9	12.1	53.7	10.4
Beans, baked, canned, w/o salt	1 cup	266	1	12.1	52.1	13.9

FOOD ITEM

FOOD ITEM	Serving Size	Cal.	Fat	Protein	Carbs	Fiber
B (cont.)						
Beans, baked, canned, w/ beef	1 cup	322	9.2	17	45	10
Beans, black, cooked	1 cup	227	0.9	15	40	15
Beans, cranberry, cooked	1 cup	241	0.8	16	43	18
Beans, fava, canned	1 cup	182	0.5	14	31	9.5
Beans, french, cooked	1 cup	228	1.3	12	43	17
Beans, great northern, cooked	1 cup	209	0.8	15	37	12
Beans, kidney, cooked	1 cup	225	0.9	15	40	11
Beans, lima, cooked	1 cup	216	0.7	15	39	13
Beans, lima, canned	1 can	190	0.4	12	36	11
Beans, mung, cooked	1 cup	212	0.7	14	39	15
Beans, mungo, cooked	1 cup	189	1	13.5	33	11.5
Beans, navy, cooked	1 cup	255	1	15	47	19
Beans, pink, cooked	1 cup	252	0.8	15	47	9
Beans, pinto, cooked	1 cup	245	1	15	44	15
Beans, small white, cooked	1 cup	254	1	16	46	18
Beans, snap, green, cooked	1 cup	44	0.3	2	10	4
Beans, snap, yellow, cooked	1 cup	44	0.3	2	10	4
Beans, white, cooked	1 cup	249	0.6	17	45	11
Beans, yellow, cooked	1 cup	255	2	16	48	18
Beechnuts, dried	1 oz	163	14.2	1.8	9.5	0
Beef ,choice short rib, cooked	3 oz	400	35.6	18.3	0	0
Beef bologna	1 slice	88	8	3.3	0.6	0
Beef jerky, chopped	1 piece	81	5.1	6.6	2.2	0.4
Beef sausage, pre-cooked	1 link	134	11.6	6	1	0
Beef stew, canned	1 serving	218	12.5	11.5	15.7	3.5
Beef, tri-tip roast, roasted	3 oz	174	9.4	22.2	0	0
Beef, brisket, lean and fat, roasted	3 oz	328	26.8	20	0	0
Beef, brisket, lean, roasted	3 oz	206	10.8	25.3	0	0
Beef, chuck ,arm roast, lean & fat, braised	3 oz	283	19.6	23.3	0	0
Beef, chuck ,arm roast, lean, braised	3 oz	179	6.5	28.1	0	0
Beef, chuck, top blade, raw	3 oz	138	7.5	16.5	0	0
Beef, cured breakfast strips	3 slices	276	26.4	8.5	0.5	0
Beef, cured, corned, canned	3 oz	213	12.8	23	0	0
Beef, cured, dried	1 serving	43	0.5	8.7	0.8	0
Beef, cured, luncheon meat	1 slice	31	0.9	5.4	0	0
Beef, flank, raw	1 oz	47	2.4	6	0	0
Beef, ground patties, frozen	3 oz	240	19.7	14.5	0	0
Beef, ground, 70% lean, raw	1 oz	94	8.5	4.1	0	0
Beef, ground, 80% lean, raw	1 oz	72	5.7	4.9	0	0
Beef, ground, 95% lean, raw	1 oz	39	1.4	6.1	0	0
Beef, rib, large end, boneless, raw	1 oz	94	8.3	4.5	0	0
Beef, rib, shortribs, boneless, raw	1 oz	110	10.3	4.1	0	0
Beef, rib, whole, boneless, raw	1 oz	91	7.9	4.6	0	0
Beef, rib-eye, small end, raw	1 oz	78	6.3	5	0	0
Beef, round, bottom, raw	1 oz	56	3.4	5.9	0	0
Beef, round, eye, raw	1 oz	49	2.5	6.1	0	0
Beef, round, full cut, raw	1 oz	55	3.4	5.8	0	0
Beef, round, tip, raw	1 oz	56	3.6	5.5	0	0
Beef, round, top, raw	1 oz	48	2.3	6.2	0	0
Beef, shank crosscuts, raw	1 oz	50	2.8	5.8	0	0

FOOD ITEM	Serving Size	Cal.	Fat	Protein	Carbs	Fiber
B (cont.)						
Beef, short loin, porterhouse, raw	1 oz	73	5.7	5.1	0	0
Beef, short loin, t-bone, raw	1 oz	66	4.8	5.4	0	0
Beef, short loin, top, raw	1 oz	66	4.5	5.8	0	0
Beef, sirloin, tri-tip, raw	1 oz	50	3	5.8	0	0
Beef, tenderloin, raw	1 oz	70	5.1	5.6	0	0
Beef, top sirloin, raw	1 oz	61	4	5.6	0	0
Beer, light	12 fl oz.	110	12	4.8	7	0
Beer, non-alcoholic	12 fl oz.	80	1	0	70	0
Beer, regular	12 fl oz.	140	12	0.9	10	0.7
Beets	1 beet	35	0	2	8	4
Bratwurst, chicken	1 serving	148	8.7	16.3	0	0
Bratwurst, pork	1 serving	281	24.8	11.7	2.1	0
Bratwurst, veal	1 serving	286	26.6	11.8	0	0
Bread stuffing, dry mix, prepared	1/2 cup	178	8.6	3	22	3
Bread, banana	1 slice	196	6.3	2.5	32.7	0.7
Bread, corn	1 piece	188	6	4.3	28.8	1.4
Bread, cracked-wheat	1 slice	65	1	2.2	11.8	1
Bread, french	1 slice	70	1	3	15	1
Bread, garlic	1 slice	160	10	3	14	1
Bread, Irish soda	1 oz	82	1.4	1.9	15.9	0.7
Bread, pita	2 oz	150	1	3	30	0
Bread, pumpernickel	1 slice	75	1	3	15	2
Bread, raisin	1 slice	80	1.5	2	15	1
Bread, rice bran	1 oz	69	1.3	2.5	12.3	1.4
Bread, sandwich slice	1 slice	70	1	2	13	1
Bread, sourdough	1 slice	100	1	2	20	1
Broadbeans, cooked	1 cup	187	0.6	13	33.4	9.2
Brownies	1 brownie	220	13	1	27	1
Buckwheat	1 cup	583	5.8	22.5	121.6	17
Buckwheat flour	1 cup	402	3.7	15.1	84.7	12
Buckwheat groats, roasted, cooked	1 cup	155	1	5.6	33.5	4.5
Buffalo, raw	1 oz	28	0.4	5.8	0	0
Burbot, raw	3 oz	77	0.7	16.4	0	0
Burdock root	1 cup	85	0.2	1.8	20.5	3.9
Butter, whipped, w/ salt	1 tbsp	67	7.6	0.1	0	0
Butternuts, dried		174	16	7	3	1.3
C						
Cabbage, common	1 cup, shredded	17	1	1	4	1.6
Cabbage, pak-choi	1 cup, shredded	9	0.1	1.1	1.5	0.7
Cabbage, pe-tsai	1 cup, shredded	12	0.2	0.9	2.5	0.9
Cake, angel food	1 slice	180	4	2	36	2
Cake, boston crème pie	1 slice	260	9	1	32	0
Cake, carrot	1 slice	310	16	1	39	0
Cake, cheesecake	1 slice	500	30	4	50	0
Cake, chocolate	1 slice	270	13	1	36	1
Cake, chocolate mousse	1 slice	250	11	1	35	1
Cake, devil's food	1 slice	270	13	2	35	0
Cake, pineapple upside-down	1 piece	367	13.9	4	58.1	0.9
Cake, pound	1 slice	320	16	2	38	0

FOOD ITEM

C (cont.)

FOOD ITEM	Serving Size	Cal.	Fat	Protein	Carbs	Fiber
Cake, sponge cake w/ cream, berries	1 slice	325	8	25	38	1
Cake, yellow	1 slice	260	11	2	36	1
Candy, butterscotch	5 pieces	120	2.5	0	20	0
Candy, caramels	1 piece	30	1	3	6	1
Candy, carob	1 bar	470	27.3	7.1	49	3.3
Candy, chocolate fudge	1 oz.	125	5	0	18	0
Candy, chocolate mints	1 mint	45	1	0	9	0
Candy, milk chocolate w/ almonds	1.5 oz.	216	14	3.7	21	2.5
Candy, chocolate-coated peanut butter bites	1 piece	45	2.5	1	4	0
Candy, chocolate-coated peanuts	12 peanuts	160	11	20	15	7
Candy, gum drops	4 pieces	130	0	0	31	0
Candy, hard candy	1 piece	18	0	0	5	0
Candy, jellybeans	12 beans	100	0	0	24	0
Candy, licorice	1 piece	30	0	0	7	0
Candy, lollipop	1 lollipop	20	0	0	5	0
Candy, milk chocolate bar	1.5 oz.	235	13	3.3	26	1.5
Candy, mints	1 mint	30	0	0	7	0
Cantaloupe	1 cup, cubed	54	0.3	1.3	13.1	1.4
Cardoon	1 cup, shredded	36	0.2	1.2	8.7	2.8
Carrots	1 medium	65	0	1	15	4
Cashew butter, w/ salt	1 tbsp	94	7.9	2.8	4.4	0.3
Cashew nuts	1 oz	157	12.4	5.2	8.6	0.9
Cassava	1 cup	330	0.6	2.8	78.4	3.7
Celeriac	1 cup	66	0.5	2.3	14.4	2.8
Chard, swiss	1 cup	7	0.1	0.6	1.3	0.6
Cheese, American	1 slice	110	9	5	1	0
Cheese, brick	1 oz.	100	8	31	0	0
Cheese, brie	1 oz.	95	8	50	1	0
Cheese, camembert	1 oz.	90	7	49	1	0
Cheese, cheddar	1 oz.	110	9	33	0.5	0
Cheese, colby-jack	1 oz.	110	9	31	0.5	0
Cheese, cottage, 2%	1 cup	203	4	31	8	0
Cheese, edam	1 oz.	100	8	7	0	0
Cheese, feta	1 oz.	100	8	21	1	0
Cheese, goat	1 oz	128	10.1	8.7	0.6	0
Cheese, goat, semi-soft	1 oz	103	8.5	6.1	0.7	0
Cheese, goat, soft	1 oz	76	6	5.3	0.3	0
Cheese, gouda	1 oz.	100	8	7	0.5	0
Cheese, monterey-jack	1 oz.	110	9	32	0	0
Cheese, mozzarella	1 oz.	90	7	25	0.5	0
Cheese, parmesan, hard	1 oz.	110	7	10	1	0
Cheese, parmesan, shredded	1 tbsp	22	1.5	2	0	0
Cheese, provolone	1 oz.	100	8	34	1	0
Cheese, queso	2 tbsp	110	9	28	2	0
Cheese, ricotta	2 tbsp	50	3.5	28	1	0
Cheese, roquefort	1 oz.	105	9	6	0.5	0
Cheese, swiss	1 oz.	110	9	36	1	0
Cherries, sour	8 pieces	30	0	1	7	2
Cherries, sweet	8 pieces	30	0	2	7	2
Chewing gum	1 piece	25	0	0	5	0

FOOD ITEM

C (cont.)

FOOD ITEM	Serving Size	Cal.	Fat	Protein	Carbs	Fiber
Chicken, breast, w/ skin	1/2 breast	249	13.4	30.2	0	0
Chicken, breast, w/o skin	1/2 breast	130	1.5	27.2	0	0
Chicken, capons, boneless	1/2 capon	1459	74	184	0	0
Chicken, capons, giblets, cooked	1 cup	238	8	38	1	0
Chicken, cornish game hen, roasted	1/2 bird	336	24	29	0	0
Chicken, cornish game hen, meat only	1 bird	295	9	51	0	0
Chicken, dark meat, w/o skin	1 cup diced	287	14	38	0	0
Chicken, drumstick, w/ skin	1 drumstick	118	6.3	14.1	0	0
Chicken, drumstick, w/o skin	1 drumstick	74	2.1	12.8	0	0
Chicken, leg, w/ skin	1 leg	312	20.2	30.3	0	0
Chicken, leg, w/o skin	1 leg	156	5	26.2	0	0
Chicken, light meat, w/o skin	1 cup diced	214	6	38	0	0
Chicken, thigh, w/ skin	1 thigh	198	14.3	16.2	0	0
Chicken, thigh, w/o skin	1 thigh	82	2.7	13.6	0	0
Chicken, wing, w/ skin	1 wing	109	7.8	9	0	0
Chicken, wing, w/o skin	1 wing	37	1	6.4	0	0
Chickpeas, cooked	1 cup	269	4	15	45	12.5
Chicory greens	1 cup, chopped	41	0.5	3.1	8.5	7.2
Chicory roots	1/2 cup	33	0.1	0.6	7.9	0
Chicory, witloof	1/2 cup	8	0	0.4	1.8	1.4
Chili con carne w/ beans	1 cup	298	13	17.5	28	10
Chili powder	1 tsp	8	0.4	0.3	1.4	0.9
Chili w/ beans, canned	1 cup	287	14	14.5	30.5	11
Chili w/o beans, canned	1 cup	194	6.5	17	18	3
Chinese chestnuts	1 oz	64	0.3	1.2	13.9	0
Chives	1 tbsp, chopped	1	0	0.1	0.1	0.1
Chocolate chip crisped rice bar	1 bar	115	3.8	1.4	20.7	0.6
Chocolate chips	1/4 cup	210	12	3	24	1
Chocolate milkshake, ready-to-drink	8 fl oz	181	5	8	26	1
Chocolate, semi-sweet bars, baking	1 oz	160	8	3	20	1
Chocolate, unsweetened baking squares	1 square	144	15	3.7	8.6	4.8
Chorizo, pork and beef	1 link	273	23	14.5	1.1	0
Chow mein noodles	1 cup	237	13.8	3.8	25.9	1.8
Cinnamon, ground	1 tsp	6	0.1	0.1	1.8	1.2
Cisco	3 oz	83	1.6	16.1	0	0
Citrus fruit drink, from concentrate	8 fl oz	124	0.1	0.5	30	0.8
Clam, mixed species, raw	1 large	15	0.2	2.6	0.5	0
Cloves, ground	1 tsp	7	0.4	0.1	1.3	0.7
Cocktail mix, non-alcoholic	1 fl oz	103	0	0.1	25.8	0
Cocoa mix, powder	1 serving	113	1.1	1.7	24	1
Cocoa mix, powder, unsweetened	1 tbsp	12	0.7	1.1	2.9	1.8
Coconut meat	1 cup, shredded	283	26.8	2.7	12.2	7.2
Coconut milk	1 cup	552	57.2	5.5	13.3	5.3
Coffee, brewed, decaf	1 cup	0	0	0.2	0	0
Coffee, brewed, regular	1 cup	2	0	0.3	0	0
Coffee, café au lait	8 fl oz.	65	2.5	1	6	0
Coffee, cappuccino	8 fl oz	70	4	1	6	0
Coffee, espresso	1 shot	4	0	0	1	0
Coffee, instant, decaf	1 tsp	0	0	0	0	0
Coffee, instant, regular	1 tsp, dry	2	0	0.1	0.4	0

FOOD ITEM

C (cont.)

FOOD ITEM	Serving Size	Cal.	Fat	Protein	Carbs	Fiber
Coffee, latte	8 fl oz.	100	5	0	8	0
Coffee, mocha	8 fl oz.	180	12	1	16	0
Coffeecake	2.5 oz.	230	7	3.8	38	3.8
Coleslaw	1/2 cup	41	1.6	0.8	7.4	0.9
Collards	1 cup, chopped	11	0.2	0.9	2	1.3
Conch, baked or broiled	1 cup, sliced	165	1.5	33.4	2.2	0
Cookies, animal crackers	1 cookie	22	0.7	0.3	3.6	0.1
Cookies, brownies	3.5 oz.	430	25	1	52	1.2
Cookies, butter	1 cookie	23	0.9	0.3	3.4	0
Cookies, chocolate chip, deli fresh baked	1 cookie	275	15	0	37.5	1
Cookies, chocolate chip, commercial	1 cookie	130	6.9	0.9	16.7	0.9
Cookies, chocolate chip, refrigerated dough	1 portion	128	5.9	1.3	17.8	0.4
Cookies, chocolate wafers	1 wafer	26	0.8	0.4	4.3	0.2
Cookies, fig bars	1 cookie	150	3.1	1.6	30.5	2
Cookies, fudge	1 cookie	73	0.8	1.1	16.4	0.6
Cookies, gingersnap	1 cookie	29	0.7	0.4	5.4	0.2
Cookies, graham, plain or honey	2 1/2" square	30	0.7	0.5	5.3	0.2
Cookies, marshmallow w/ chocolate coating	1 cookie	118	4.7	1.1	19	0.6
Cookies, molasses	1 cookie	138	4.1	1.8	23.6	0.3
Cookies, oatmeal	1 cookie	238	8.8	2.5	37.5	2
Cookies, oatmeal w/ raisins	1 cookie	238	8.8	2.5	37.5	2
Cookies, oatmeal, commercial, iced	1 cookie	123	4.8	1.4	18.4	0.6
Cookies, oatmeal, refrigerated dough	1 portion	68	3	0.9	9.5	0.4
Cookies, peanut butter sandwich	1 cookie	67	3	1.2	9.2	0.3
Cookies, peanut butter, refrigerated dough	1 portion	73	4	1.3	8.3	0.2
Cookies, sugar	1 cookie	66	3.3	0.8	8.4	0.2
Cookies, sugar wafers w/ cream filling	1 wafer	46	2.2	0.4	6.3	0.1
Cookies, sugar, refrigerated dough	1 portion	113	5.4	1.1	15.3	0.2
Cookies, vanilla wafers	1 wafer	28	1.2	0.3	4.3	0.1
Coriander leaves	9 sprigs	5	0.1	0.4	0.7	0.6
Corn flour, yellow	1 cup	416	4.3	10.6	86.9	0
Corn, sweet, white	1 ear	77	1.1	2.9	17.1	2.4
Corn, sweet, yellow	1 ear	77	1.1	2.9	17.1	2.4
Corn, sweet, white, cream style	1 cup	184	1	4.5	46.4	3.1
Corn, sweet, yellow, cream style	1 cup	184	1	4.5	46.4	3.1
Cornnuts	1 oz	126	4.4	2.4	20.4	2
Cornstarch	1 cup	488	0.1	0.3	116.8	1.2
Couscous, cooked	1 cup	176	0.2	6	36.5	0
Cowpeas (blackeyes), cooked	1 cup	160	0.6	5.2	33.5	8.2
Cowpeas, cat jang, cooked	1 cup	200	1.2	14	34.7	6.2
Cowpeas, leafy tips	1 cup, chopped	10	0.1	1.5	1.7	0
Crab, Alaska king, raw	1 leg	144	1	31.5	0	0
Crab, blue, canned	1 cup	134	1.6	27.7	0	0
Crab, dungeness, cooked	1 crab	140	1.6	28.4	1.2	0
Crabapples	1 cup, sliced	84	0.3	0.4	21.9	0
Crackers w/ cheese filling	6 crackers	191	9.5	3.5	22.9	0.7
Crackers w/ peanut butter filling	6 crackers	193	9.8	4.8	22.1	1.3
Crackers, cheese, regular	6 crackers	312	15.7	6.3	36.1	1.5
Crackers, graham	1 cracker	30	0.5	6	5	2
Crackers, matzo, plain	1 matzo	112	0.4	2.8	23.7	0.9

FOOD ITEM

FOOD ITEM	Serving Size	Cal.	Fat	Protein	Carbs	Fiber

C (cont.)

FOOD ITEM	Serving Size	Cal.	Fat	Protein	Carbs	Fiber
Crackers, matzo, whole-wheat	1 matzo	100	0.4	3.7	22.4	3.3
Crackers, melba toast	1 cup	129	1.1	4	25.3	2.1
Crackers, milk	1 cracker	50	1.7	0.8	7.7	0.2
Crackers, regular	1 cup, bite size	311	15.7	4.6	37.8	1
Crackers, rusk toast	1 rusk	41	0.7	1.4	7.2	0
Crackers, rye	1 cracker	37	0.1	1.1	8.8	2.5
Crackers, saltines	1 cracker	20	0.1	0.5	4.1	0.1
Crackers, soda	1 cracker	60	2	6	10	2
Crackers, wheat	1 cracker	9	0.4	0.1	1.3	0.1
Crackers, wheat, sandwich w/ peanut butter	1 cracker	35	1.8	0.9	3.7	0.3
Crackers, whole-wheat	1 cracker	18	0.7	0.3	2.7	0.4
Cranberries	1 cup, whole	44	0.1	0.4	11.6	4.4
Cranberry juice cocktail	1 cup	144	0.3	0	36.4	0.3
Cranberry-apple juice	1 cup	174	0.1	0.2	44.3	0.2
Cranberry-grape juice	1 cup	137	0.2	0.5	34.3	0.2
Crayfish, wild, raw	8 crayfish	21	0.3	4.3	0	0
Cream cheese	1 tbsp	51	5.1	1.1	0.4	0
Cream of tartar	1 tsp	8	0	0	1.8	0
Cream, half & half	1 tbsp	20	1.7	0.4	0.6	0
Cream, heavy whipping	1 cup, fluid	821	88.1	4.9	6.6	0
Crepes	1 crepe	120	6	2	14	1
Croissants, apple	1 croissant	145	5	4.2	21.1	1.4
Croissants, butter	1 croissant	115	6	2.3	13	0.7
Croissants, cheese	1 croissant	174	8.8	3.9	19.7	1.1
Croutons, plain	1 cup	122	2	3.6	22.1	1.5
Croutons, seasoned	1 cup	186	7.3	4.3	25.4	2
Cucumber	1 cucumber	45	0.3	2	10.9	1.5
Cucumber, peeled	1 cup, sliced	14	0.2	0.7	2.6	0.8
Cumin seed	1 tsp	8	0.5	0.4	0.9	0.2
Currants, black	1 cup	71	0.5	1.6	17.2	0
Currants, red & white	1 cup	63	0.2	1.6	15.5	4.8
Curry powder	1 tsp	7	0.3	0.3	1.2	0.7

D

FOOD ITEM	Serving Size	Cal.	Fat	Protein	Carbs	Fiber
Dandelion greens	1 cup, chopped	25	0.4	1.5	5.1	1.9
Danish pastry, cheese, 4 1/4" diameter	1 pastry	266	15.5	5.7	26.4	0.7
Danish pastry, cinnamon, 4 1/4" diameter	1 pastry	262	14.5	4.5	29	0.8
Danish pastry, fruit, 4 1/4" diameter	1 pastry	263	13	3.8	33.9	1.3
Danish pastry, nut, 4 1/4" diameter	1 pastry	280	16.4	4.6	29.7	1.3
Danish pastry, raspberry, 4 1/4" diameter	1 pastry	263	13.1	3.8	33.9	1.3
Deer, ground, raw	1 oz	45	2	6.2	0	0
Deer, raw	1 oz	34	0.7	6.5	0	0
Doughnuts, chocolate coated or frosted	1 doughnut	133	8.7	1.4	13.4	0.6
Doughnuts, chocolate, sugared or glazed	1 doughnut	250	11.9	2.7	34.4	1.3
Doughnuts, french crullers	1 cruller	169	7.5	1.3	24.4	0.5
Doughnuts, plain	1 doughnut, stick	219	11.9	2.6	25.8	0.8
Doughnuts, wheat, sugared or glazed	1 doughnut	101	5.4	1.8	11.9	0.6
Duck liver, raw	1 liver	60	2	8.2	1.6	0
Duck, meat only, roasted	1/2 duck	444	24.7	51.9	0	0
Duck, white pekin, breast w/skin. roasted	1/2 breast	242	13	29.4	0	0

264

FOOD ITEM	Serving Size	Cal.	Fat	Protein	Carbs	Fiber
D (cont.)						
Duck, skinless, raw	1/2 duck	400	18	55.4	0	0
Durian	1 cup, chopped	357	13	3.6	65.8	9.2
E						
Eclairs w/ chocolate glaze	1 éclair	293	17.6	7.2	27.1	0.7
Eel, mixed species, raw	3 oz	156	9.9	15.7	0	0
Egg noodles, cooked	1 cup	213	2.3	7.6	39.7	1.8
Egg substitute, liquid	1 tbsp	13	0.5	1.9	0.1	0
Egg white, fried	1 large	92	7	6.3	0.4	0
Egg white, raw	1 large	17	0.1	3.6	0.2	0
Egg yolk, raw	1 large	53	4.4	2.6	0.6	0
Egg, hard-boiled	1 cup, chopped	211	14.4	17.1	1.5	0
Egg, omelette	1 large	93	7.3	6.5	0.4	0
Egg, poached	1 large	74	4.9	6.3	0.4	0
Egg, raw	1 large	85	5.8	7.3	0.4	0
Egg, scrambled	1 cup	365	26.9	24.4	4.8	0
Eggnog	8 fl oz	343	19	9.6	34	0
Eggplant	1 eggplant	110	0.9	4.6	26.1	15.6
Elderberries	1 cup	106	0.7	1	26.7	10.2
Elk, ground, raw	1 oz	49	2.5	6.2	0	0
Elk, raw	1 oz	31	0.4	6.5	0	0
Endive	1 head	87	1	6.4	17.2	15.9
English muffins, plain	1 muffin	134	1	4.4	26.2	1.5
English muffins, cinnamon-raisin	1 muffin	139	1.5	4.2	48.7	1.7
English muffins, wheat	1 muffin	127	1.1	5	25.5	2.6
English muffins, whole-wheat	1 muffin	134	1.4	5.8	26.6	4.4
English muffins, whole-wheat/multi-grain	1 muffin	155	1.2	6	30.5	1.8
European chestnuts, peeled	1 oz	56	0.4	0.5	12.5	0
European chestnuts, unpeeled	1 oz	60	0.6	0.7	12.9	2.3
F						
Farina, cooked	1 cup	471	0.1	3.3	24.4	0.7
Fast Food, biscuit w/ egg	1 biscuit	373	22.1	11.6	31.9	0.8
Fast Food, biscuit w/ egg & bacon	1 biscuit	458	31.1	17	28.6	0.8
Fast Food, biscuit w/ egg, bacon & cheese	1 biscuit	477	31.4	16.3	33.4	0.1
Fast Food, biscuit w/ sausage	1 biscuit	485	31.8	12.1	40	1.4
Fast Food, caramel sundae	1 sundae	304	9.3	7.3	49.3	0
Fast Food, cheeseburger, large, double patty	1 sandwich	704	43.7	38	39.7	1
Fast Food, cheeseburger, large, single patty	1 sandwich	563	32.9	28.2	38.4	1
Fast Food, corndog	1 corndog	460	18.9	16.8	55.8	1
Fast Food, croissant w/ egg, cheese	1 croissant	368	24.7	12.8	24.3	1
Fast Food, croissant w/ egg, cheese, bacon	1 croissant	413	28.4	16.2	23.6	1
Fast Food, croissant w/ egg, cheese, sausage	1 croissant	523	38.2	20.3	24.7	1
Fast Food, Danish pastry, cheese	1 pastry	353	24.6	5.8	28.7	1.5
Fast Food, Danish pastry, cinnamon	1 pastry	349	16.7	4.8	46.9	1.5
Fast Food, Danish pastry, fruit	1 pastry	335	15.9	4.8	45.1	1.5
Fast Food, fish sandwich w/ tartar sauce	1 sandwich	431	22.8	16.9	41	1
Fast Food, french toast sticks	5 pieces	513	29	8.3	57.9	2.7
Fast Food, fried chicken, boneless	6 pieces	285	18.1	15	15.7	0.9
Fast Food, hamburger, large, double patty	1 sandwich	540	26.6	34.3	40.3	2.1

FOOD ITEM

	Serving Size	Cal.	Fat	Protein	Carbs	Fiber

F (cont.)

FOOD ITEM	Serving Size	Cal.	Fat	Protein	Carbs	Fiber
Fast Food, hamburger, large, single patty	1 sandwich	425	20.9	23	36.7	2.1
Fast Food, hot fudge sundae	1 sundae	284	8.6	5.6	47.7	0
Fast Food, hot dog w/ chili	1 hot dog	296	13.4	13.5	31.3	1
Fast Food, hot dog, plain	1 hot dog	242	14.5	10.4	18	1
Fast Food, McDonald's Big Mac® w/ cheese	1 serving	560	30	25	46	3.1
Fast Food, McDonald's Big Mac® w/o cheese	1 serving	495	25.4	23.2	43.3	2.7
Fast Food, McDonald's cheeseburger	1 serving	310	12	15	35	1
Fast Food, McDonald's Chicken McGrill®	1 serving	400	16	27	38	3
Fast Food, McDonald's Crispy Chicken	1 serving	500	23	24	50	3
Fast Food, McDonald's Filet-o-Fish®	1 serving	400	18	14	42	1
Fast Food, McDonald's french fries	1 medium	350	11	4	47	5
Fast Food, McDonald's hamburger	1 serving	260	9	13	33	1
Fast Food, McDonald's 1/4 Pounder®,cheese	1 serving	510	25	29	43	3
Fast Food, McDonald's 1/4 Pounder®	1 serving	420	18	24	40	3
Fast Food, onion rings, 8-9 rings	1 portion	276	15.5	3.7	31.3	3.3
Fast Food, strawberry sundae	1 sundae	268	7.8	6.3	44.6	0
Fast Food, submarine sandwich w/ cold cuts	1 submarine 6"	456	18.6	21.8	51	4
Fast Food, submarine sandwich w/ roast beef	1 submarine 6"	410	13	28.6	44.3	4
Fast Food, submarine sandwich w/ tuna	1 submarine 6"	584	28	29.7	55.4	4
Fast Food, vanilla soft-serve w/ cone	1 cone	164	6.1	3.9	24.1	0.1
Fennel bulb	1 cup, sliced	27	0.2	1.1	6.3	2.7
Fennel seed	1 tbsp	20	0.9	0.9	3	2.3
Fenugreek seed	1 tbsp	36	0.7	2.6	6.5	2.7
Figs	1 medium	37	0.2	0.4	9.6	1.5
Figs, dried	1 fig	21	0.01	0.3	5.3	0.8
Fireweed leaves	1 cup, chopped	24	0.6	1.1	4.4	2.4
Fish oil, cod liver	1 tbsp	123	13.6	0	0	0
Fish oil, herring	1 tbsp	123	13.6	0	0	0
Fish oil, menhaden	1 tbsp	123	13.6	0	0	0
Fish oil, salmon	1 tbsp	123	13.6	0	0	0
Fish oil, sardine	1 tbsp	123	13.6	0	0	0
Fish, bluefin tuna, raw	3 oz	122	4.2	19.8	0	0
Fish, bluefish, raw	3 oz	105	3.6	17	0	0
Fish, butterfish, raw	3 oz	124	6.8	14.7	0	0
Fish, carp, raw	3 oz	108	4.8	15.2	0	0
Fish, catfish, raw	3 oz	81	2.4	13.9	0	0
Fish, cod, atlantic, raw	3 oz	70	0.6	15.1	0	0
Fish, croaker, atlantic, raw	3 oz	88	2.7	15.1	0	0
Fish, flatfish, raw	3 oz	77	1	16	0	0
Fish, gefilte fish	1 piece	35	0.7	3.8	3.1	0
Fish, grouper, mixed species, raw	3 oz	78	0.9	16.5	0	0
Fish, haddock, raw	3 oz	74	0.6	16.1	0	0
Fish, halibut, raw	3 oz	94	1.9	17.7	0	0
Fish, herring, atlantic, raw	3 oz	134	7.7	15.3	0	0
Fish, herring, pacific, raw	3 oz	166	11.8	13.9	0	0
Fish, mackerel, atlantic, raw	3 oz	174	11.8	15.8	0	0
Fish, mackerel, king, raw	3 oz	89	1.7	17.2	0	0
Fish, mackerel, pacific, raw	3 oz	134	6.7	17.1	0	0
Fish, mackerel, spanish, raw	3 oz	118	5.4	16.4	0	0
Fish, milkfish, raw	3 oz	126	5.7	17.5	0	0

FOOD ITEM

FOOD ITEM	Serving Size	Cal.	Fat	Protein	Carbs	Fiber
F (cont.)						
Fish, monkfish, raw	3 oz	65	1.3	12.3	0	0
Fish, ocean perch, atlantic, raw	3 oz	80	1.4	15.8	0	0
Fish, perch, mixed species, raw	3 oz	77	0.8	16.5	0	0
Fish, pike, northern, raw	3 oz	75	0.6	16.4	0	0
Fish, pollock, atlantic, raw	3 oz	78	0.8	16.5	0	0
Fish, pout, ocean, raw	3 oz	67	0.8	14.1	0	0
Fish, rainbow smelt, raw	3 oz	82	2.1	15	0	0
Fish, rockfish, pacific, raw	3 oz	80	1.3	15.9	0	0
Fish, roe, mixed species, raw	1 tbsp	20	0.9	3.1	0.2	0
Fish, sablefish, raw	3 oz	166	13	11.4	0	0
Fish, salmon, atlantic, farmed, raw	3 oz	156	9.2	16.9	0	0
Fish, salmon, atlantic, wild, raw	3 oz	121	5.4	16.9	0	0
Fish, salmon, chinook, raw	3 oz	152	8.9	16.9	0	0
Fish, salmon, pink, raw	3 oz	99	2.9	16.9	0	0
Fish, sea bass, mixed species, raw	3 oz	82	1.7	15.7	0	0
Fish, seatrout, mixed species, raw	3 oz	88	3.1	14.2	0	0
Fish, shad, raw	3 oz	167	11.7	14.4	0	0
Fish, skipjack tuna, raw	3 oz	88	0.9	18.7	0	0
Fish, snapper, mixed species, raw	3 oz	85	1.1	17.4	0	0
Fish, striped bass, raw	3 oz	82	2	15.1	0	0
Fish, striped mullet, raw	3 oz	99	3.2	16.4	0	0
Fish, sturgeon, mixed species, raw	3 oz	89	3.4	13.7	0	0
Fish, swordfish, raw	3 oz	103	3.4	16.8	0	0
Fish, trout, mixed species, raw	3 oz	126	5.6	17.7	0	0
Fish, white sucker, raw	3 oz	78	2	14.2	0	0
Fish, whitefish, raw	3 oz	114	5	16.2	0	0
Fish, wolffish, atlantic, raw	3 oz	82	2	14.9	0	0
Fish, yellowfin tuna, raw	3 oz	93	0.9	19.8	0	0
Fish, yellowtail, mixed species, raw	3 oz	124	4.5	19.7	0	0
Flan, caramel custard	5 1/2 oz.	303	12	4	43	0
Flaxseed	1 tbsp	59	4.1	2.3	4.1	3.3
Flaxseed oil	1 tbsp	120	13.6	0	0	0
Frankfurter	1 serving	151	13.4	5.3	2.2	0
Frankfurter, beef	1 frankfurter	188	16.9	6.4	2.3	0
Frankfurter, beef & pork	1 frankfurter	174	15.8	6.6	1	1.4
Frankfurter, chicken	1 frankfurter	116	8.8	5.8	3.1	0
Frankfurter, meat	1 frankfurter	151	13.4	5.3	2.2	0
Frankfurter, meatless	1 frankfurter	163	9.6	13.7	5.4	2.7
Frankfurter, pork	1 frankfurter	204	18	9.7	0.2	0.1
Frankfurter, turkey	1 frankfurter	102	8	6.4	0.7	0
French fries, frozen, unprepared, 18 fries	1 serving	170	6.7	2.8	27.7	3.4
French toast , frozen, ready-to-heat	1 piece	126	3.6	4.3	18.9	0.6
Frosting, creamy chocolate	2 tbsp	164	7.3	0.5	26.1	0.4
Frosting, creamy vanilla	2 tbsp	160	6.3	0	25.6	0
Frozen yogurt, chocolate, soft-serve	1/2 cup	115	4.3	2.9	17.9	1.6
Frozen yogurt, vanilla, soft-serve	1/2 cup	117	4	2.9	17.4	0
Fruit cocktail, canned	1 cup	229	0.2	1	59.5	2.9
Fruit punch, prepared from concentrate	8 fl oz.	124	0.5	0.2	30.2	0.2
Fruit salad, canned in syrup	1 cup	186	0.2	0.9	48.7	2.6
Fruit salad, canned in water	1 cup	74	0.2	0.9	19.3	2.5

FOOD ITEM

FOOD ITEM	Serving Size	Cal.	Fat	Protein	Carbs	Fiber
G						
Garden cress, raw	1 cup	16	0.3	1.3	2.7	0.6
Garlic	1 clove	4	0	0.2	1	0.1
Garlic powder	1 tsp	9	0	0.5	2	0.3
Gelatin dessert mix, prepared w/ water	1/2 cup	84	0	1.6	19.1	0
Gin, 80 Proof	1 fl oz.	73	0	0	0	0
Ginger root	1 tsp	2	0	0	0.4	0
Ginger, ground	1 tsp	6	0.1	0.2	1.3	0.2
Ginkgo nuts	1 oz	52	0.5	1.2	10.7	0
Ginkgo nuts, dried	1 oz	99	0.6	2.9	20.5	0
Goose liver, raw	1 liver	125	4	15.4	5.9	0
Goose, meat & skin, roasted	1 cup chopped	427	30.7	35.2	0	0
Goose, meat only, roasted	1 cup chopped	340	18.1	41.4	0	0
Gourd, white-flowered	1 gourd	108	0.2	4.8	26.1	0
Granola bars, hard, plain	1 bar	134	5.6	2.9	18.3	1.5
Granola bars, soft, plain	1 bar	126	4.9	2.1	19.1	1.3
Grape juice	8 fl oz.	160	0	0	40	0
Grapefruit	1/2 fruit	50	0	1	12	3
Grapefruit juice, sweetened	8 fl oz.	125	0	0	32.6	0
Grapefruit juice, unsweetened	8 fl oz.	91	0.2	1.2	21.5	0
Grapes, canned, heavy syrup	1 cup	187	0.3	1.2	50.3	1.5
Grapes, red or green	1 cup	106	0.2	1.1	27.9	1.4
Gravy mushroom, canned	1 can	149	8.1	3.8	16.3	1.2
Gravy, au jus, canned	1 can	48	0.6	3.6	7.5	0
Gravy, beef, canned	1 can	154	6.9	10.9	14	1.2
Gravy, chicken, canned	1 can	235	17	5.8	16.2	1.2
Gravy, turkey, canned	1 can	152	6.2	7.7	15.2	1.2
Guacamole dip	2 tbsp	50	4	12	4	0
Guavas	1 fruit	37	0.5	1.4	7.8	3
H						
Ham, chopped	1 slice	50	2.9	4.6	1.2	0
Ham, minced	1 slice	55	4.3	3.4	0.4	0
Ham, sliced	1 slice	46	2.4	4.6	1.1	0.4
Hazlenuts, dry roasted	1 oz.	183	17.7	4.2	5	2.7
Hazlenuts, blanched	1 oz	178	17.3	3.9	4.8	3.1
Hominy, canned, white	1 cup	119	1.5	2.4	23.5	4.1
Hominy, canned, yellow	1 cup	115	1.4	2.4	22.8	4
Honey	1 tbsp	64	0	0.1	17.3	0
Honeydew melons	1 cup, diced	61	0.2	0.9	15.5	1.4
Horseradish	1 tsp	2	0	0.1	0.6	0.2
Hot chocolate	8 fl oz.	200	10	9	25	3
Hummus	1 tbsp	23	1.3	1.1	2	0.8
Hush puppies	1 hush puppy	74	2.9	1.7	10.1	0.6
I						
Ice cream cone, rolled or sugar type	1 cone	40	0.4	0.8	8.4	0.2
Ice cream cone, wafer or cake type	1 cone	17	0.3	0.3	3.2	0.1
Ice cream, chocolate	1/2 cup	143	7.3	2.5	18.6	0.8
Ice cream, strawberry	1/2 cup	127	5.5	2.1	18.2	0.6
Ice cream, vanilla	1/2 cup	144	7.9	2.5	16.9	0.5

FOOD ITEM	Serving Size	Cal.	Fat	Protein	Carbs	Fiber
I (cont.)						
Iced tea, pre-sweetened	8 fl oz.	100	0	0	25	0
Iced tea, unsweetened	8 fl oz.	2	0	0	0	0
Italian seasoning	1 tsp	4	0	0	1	0
J						
Jams and preserves	1 tbsp	56	0	0.1	13.8	0.2
Japanese chestnuts	1 oz	44	0.2	0.6	9.9	0
Japanese soba noodles, cooked	1 cup	113	0.1	5.7	24.4	1.7
Japanese ramen noodles, packaged, dry	1 serving	195	7.3	4	28	1
Jellies	1 tbsp	55	0	0	14.4	0.2
K						
Kale	1 cup, chopped	34	0.5	2.2	6.7	1.3
Kiwifruit	1 medium	45	0	2	11	5
Kumquats	1 fruit	13	0.2	0.4	3	1.2
L						
Lamb, cubed, raw	1 oz	38	1.5	5.7	0	0
Lamb, foreshank, raw	1 oz	57	3.8	5.4	0	0
Lamb, ground, raw	1 oz	80	6.6	4.7	0	0
Lamb, leg, shank half, raw	1 oz	52	3.3	5.4	0	0
Lamb, leg, sirloin half, raw	1 oz	74	5.9	4.9	0	0
Lamb, leg, whole, choice, raw	1 oz	65	4.8	5.1	0	0
Lamb, loin, choice, raw	1 oz	79	6.4	4.9	0	0
Lamb, rib, choice, raw	1 oz	97	8.7	4.3	0	0
Lamb, shoulder, arm, raw	1 oz	69	5.4	4.9	0	0
Lamb, shoulder, blade, raw	1 oz	69	5.4	4.8	0	0
Lamb, shoulder, whole, raw	1 oz	69	5.4	4.8	0	0
Lard	1 tbsp	115	12.8	0	0	0
Leeks	1 leek	54	0.3	1.3	12.6	1.6
Lemon juice	1 cup	61	0	0.9	21.1	1
Lemon juice, canned or bottled	1 tbsp	3	0	0.1	1	0.1
Lemon pepper seasoning	1 tsp	7	0	0	1	0
Lemonade powder	1 scoop	102	0	0	26.9	0
Lemonade, pink concentrate, prepared	8 fl oz.	99	0	0.2	25.9	0
Lemonade, white concentrate, prepared	8 fl oz.	131	0.1	0.2	34	0.2
Lemons w/ peel	1 fruit	22	0.3	1.3	11.6	5.1
Lentils, cooked	1 cup	230	0.7	17.8	39.8	15.6
Lentils, sprouted, raw	1 cup	82	0.4	6.9	17	0
Lettuce, green leaf	1 cup, shredded	5	0.1	0.5	1	0.5
Lettuce, iceberg	1 cup, shredded	10	0.1	0.7	2.2	0.9
Lettuce, red leaf	1 cup, shredded	3	0	0.2	0.4	0.2
Lettuce, romaine	1 cup, shredded	8	0.1	0.6	1.5	1
Lime juice	1 cup	62	0.2	1	20.7	1
Limes	1 fruit	20	0.1	0.5	7.1	1.9
Liverwurst, pork	1 slice	59	5.1	2.5	0.4	0
Lobster, northern, raw	1 lobster	135	1.3	28.2	0.8	0
Luncheon meat, beef, loaved	1 oz.	87	7.4	4.1	0.8	0
Luncheon meat, beef, thin sliced	1 oz.	50	1.1	8	1.6	0
Luncheon meat, meatless slices	1 slice	26	1.6	2.5	0.6	0

FOOD ITEM

	Serving Size	Cal.	Fat	Protein	Carbs	Fiber
L (cont.)						
Luncheon meat, pork & chicken, minced	1 oz	56	3.9	4.3	0.4	0
Luncheon meat, pork & ham, minced	1 oz	88	7.45	3.75	1.3	0
Luncheon meat, pork or beef	1 oz.	99	9	3.5	0.6	0
Luncheon meat, pork, canned	1 oz.	95	8.6	3.5	0.6	0
Luncheon meat, pork, ham & chicken, minced	1 oz	87	7.6	3.7	0.8	0
Luncheon sausage, pork & beef	1 oz.	74	5.9	4.3	0.4	0
M						
Macadamia nuts	1 oz. (10-12 nuts)	203	21.5	2.2	3.6	2.3
Macaroni and cheese, commercial, prepared	1 cup	259	2.6	11.3	47.5	1.5
Macaroni, cooked	1 cup	197	0.9	6.6	39.6	1.8
Malt drink mix, dry	3 heaping tsp	87	1.7	2.4	15.9	0.2
Malt beverage	8 fl oz.	144	0.2	0.7	32.2	0
Mangos	1 fruit	135	0.6	1.1	35.2	3.7
Maraschino cherries	1 cherry	8	0	0	2.1	0.2
Margarine, fat-free spread	1 tbsp	6	0.4	0	0.6	0
Margarine, stick	1 tbsp	100	11.2	0	0.3	0
Margarine, stick, unsalted	1 tbsp	102	11.4	0.1	0.1	0
Margarine, tub	1 tbsp	102	11.4	0.1	0.1	0
Martini	1 fl oz	69	0	0	0.6	0
Mayonnaise	1 tbsp	100	11	0	0.1	0
Milk, 1% low fat	1 cup	102	2.4	8.2	12.2	0
Milk, 2% low fat	1 cup	138	4.9	9.7	13.5	0
Milk, buttermilk, cultured, reduced fat	1 cup	137	4.9	10	13	0
Milk, chocolate	1 cup	208	8.5	7.9	25.9	2
Milk, dry, non fat, instant	1/3 cup dry	82	0.1	8	12	0
Milk, evaporated	1/2 cup	169	9.5	8.5	12.6	0
Milk, skim or nonfat	1 cup	83	0.2	8.5	12.2	0
Milk, canned, sweetened condensed	1 cup	982	26.6	24.2	166.5	0
Milk, whole	1 cup	146	7.9	7.9	11	0
Milkshake dry mix, vanilla	1 envelope packet	69	0.5	4.9	11.1	0.3
Millet	1 cup	756	8.4	22	145.7	17
Miso soup	1 cup	547	16.5	32.1	72.8	14.9
Mixed nuts	1 cup	814	70.5	23.7	34.7	12.3
Molasses	1 tablespoon	58	0	0	15	0
Muffins, apple bran	1 muffin	300	3	1	61	1
Muffins, banana nut	1 muffin	480	24	3	60	2
Muffins, blueberry	1 muffin	313	7.3	6.2	54.2	2.9
Muffins, chocolate chip	1 muffin	510	24	2	69	4
Muffins, corn	1 muffin	345	9.5	6.6	57.5	3.8
Muffins, oat-bran	1 muffin	305	8.3	7.9	54.5	5.2
Muffins, plain	1 muffin	242	9.1	3.8	36.3	1.5
Mushrooms	1 cup, pieces	15	0.2	2.2	2.3	0.8
Mushrooms, enoki	1 large	2	0	0.1	0.4	0.1
Mushrooms, oyster	1 large	55	0.8	6.1	9.2	3.6
Mushrooms, portobello	1 large	0	0	0	0	0
Mushrooms, shiitake	1 mushroom	11	0	0.3	2.7	0.4
Mussel, blue, raw	1 cup	129	3.4	17.8	5.5	0
Mustard greens	1 cup, chopped	15	0.1	1.5	2.7	1.8
Mustard seed, yellow	1 tbsp	53	3.2	2.8	3.9	1.6

FOOD ITEM	Serving Size	Cal.	Fat	Protein	Carbs	Fiber
M (cont.)						
Mustard spinach	1 cup, chopped	33	0.5	3.3	5.9	4.2
Mustard, prepared, yellow	1 tsp	3	0.2	0.2	0.4	0.2
N						
Natto (fermented soybeans)	1 cup	371	19.3	31	25.1	9.5
Nectarines	1 fruit	60	0.4	1.4	14.3	2.3
New Zealand spinach	1 cup, chopped	8	0.1	0.8	1.4	0
Nutmeg, ground	1 tsp	12	0.8	0.1	1.1	0.5
O						
Oat bran	1 cup	231	6.6	16.3	62.2	14.5
Oatmeal, instant, prepared w/ water	1 cup	129	2.1	5.4	22.4	3.7
Oil, canola & corn	1 tbsp	124	14	0	0	0
Oil, canola & soybean	1 tbsp	120	13.6	0	0	0
Oil, coconut	1 tbsp	120	13.6	0	0	0
Oil, corn, peanut & olive	1 tbsp	120	13.6	0	0	0
Oil, olive	1 tbsp	119	13.5	0	0	0
Oil, peanut	1 tbsp	119	13.5	0	0	0
Oil, sesame	1 tbsp	120	13.6	0	0	0
Oil, soy	1 tbsp	120	13.6	0	0	0
Oil, vegetable, almond	1 tbsp	120	13.6	0	0	0
Oil, vegetable, cocoa butter	1 tbsp	120	13.6	0	0	0
Oil, vegetable, coconut	1 tbsp	117	13.6	0	0	0
Oil, vegetable, grapeseed	1 tbsp	120	13.6	0	0	0
Oil, vegetable, hazelnut	1 tbsp	120	13.6	0	0	0
Oil, vegetable, nutmeg butter	1 tbsp	120	13.6	0	0	0
Oil, vegetable, palm	1 tbsp	120	13.6	0	0	0
Oil, vegetable, poppyseed	1 tbsp	120	13.6	0	0	0
Oil, vegetable, rice bran	1 tbsp	120	13.6	0	0	0
Oil, vegetable, sheanut	1 tbsp	120	13.6	0	0	0
Oil, vegetable, tomatoseed	1 tbsp	120	13.6	0	0	0
Oil, vegetable, walnut	1 tbsp	1927	218	0	0	0
Okra	1 cup	31	0.1	2	7	3.2
Onion powder	1 tsp	8	0	0.2	1.9	0.1
Onions	1 cup, chopped	67	0.1	1.5	16.2	2.2
Onions, sweet	1 onion	106	0.3	2.7	25	3
Orange juice	8 fl oz	109	0.6	1.9	25	0.5
Orange marmalade	1 tbsp	49	0	0.1	13.3	0.1
Oranges	1 large	86	0.2	1.7	21.6	4.4
Oregano, dried	1 tsp, ground	6	0.2	0.2	1.2	0.8
Oyster, eastern, raw	3 oz.	50	1.3	4.4	4.6	0
Oyster, pacific, raw	3 oz.	69	1.9	8	4.2	0
P						
Pancakes, blueberry	1 pancake	84	3.5	2.3	11	0
Pancakes, buttermilk	1 pancake	86	3.5	2.6	10.9	0
Pancakes, plain, dry mix	1 pancake	74	1	2	13.9	0.5
Papayas	1 cup, cubed	55	0.2	0.9	13.7	2.5
Paprika	1 tsp	6	0.3	0.3	1.2	0.8
Parsley	1 cup	22	0.5	1.8	3.8	2

FOOD ITEM

FOOD ITEM	Serving Size	Cal.	Fat	Protein	Carbs	Fiber
P (cont.)						
Parsley, dried	1 tsp	1	0	0.1	0.2	0.1
Parsnips	1 cup, sliced	100	0.4	1.6	23.9	6.5
Passion-fruit	1 fruit	17	0.1	0.4	4.2	1.9
Pasta, corn, cooked	1 cup	176	1	3.6	39	6.7
Pasta, plain, cooked	1 cup	197	0.9	6.6	39.6	2.4
Pasta, spinach, cooked	1 cup	195	1.4	7.6	37.5	2.4
Pastrami, turkey	1 oz	40	1.8	5.2	0.5	0
Pate de foie gras	1 tbsp	60	5.7	1.5	0.6	0
Pate, chicken liver, canned	1 tbsp	26	1.7	1.7	0.9	0
Pate, goose liver, canned	1 tbsp	60	5.7	1.5	0.6	0
Peaches	1 large	61	0.4	1.4	15	2.4
Peaches, canned	1 cup, halved	59	0.1	1.1	14.9	3.2
Peanut butter, chunky	2 tbsp	188	16	7.7	6.9	2.6
Peanut butter, smooth	2 tbsp	188	16.1	8	6.3	1.9
Peanuts, dry roasted w/ salt	1 oz	166	14	6.7	6.1	2.3
Peanuts, raw	1 oz	161	13.9	7.3	4.5	2.4
Pears	1 pear	121	0.3	0.8	32.3	6.5
Pears, asian	1 pear	116	0.6	1.4	29.3	9.9
Pears, canned	1 cup	71	0.1	0.5	19.1	3.9
Peas, green, fresh, cooked	1 cup	134	0.3	8.5	25	8.8
Peas, green, frozen, cooked	1 cup	125	0.4	8.2	22.8	8.8
Peas, split, cooked	1 cup	231	0.7	16.3	41.3	16.3
Pecans	1 oz. (20 halves)	196	20.4	2.6	3.9	2.7
Pepper, black	1 tsp	5	0.1	0.2	1.4	0.6
Pepper, red or cayenne	1 tsp	6	0.3	0.2	1	0.5
Pepperoni	15 slices	135	11.7	5.9	1.2	0.4
Peppers, chili, green	1 cup	29	0.4	1	6.4	2.4
Peppers, chili, red	1 pepper	18	0.2	0.8	4	0.7
Peppers, chili, sun-dried	1 pepper	2	0	0.1	0.4	0.2
Peppers, jalapeno	1 pepper	4	0.1	0.2	0.8	0.4
Peppers, sweet, green	1 medium	24	0.2	1	5.5	2
Peppers, sweet, red	1 medium	31	0.3	1.1	7.2	2.4
Peppers, sweet, yellow	1 medium	32	0.2	1.2	7.5	1.1
Persimmons	1 fruit	32	0.1	0.2	8.4	0
Pheasant, boneless, raw	1/2 pheasant	724	37.2	90.8	0	0
Pheasant, breast, skinless, boneless, raw	1/2 breast	242	5.9	44.4	0	0
Pheasant, leg, skinless, boneless, raw	1 leg	143	4.6	23.8	0	0
Pheasant, skinless, raw	1/2 pheasant	468	12.8	83	0	0
Pickle relish, sweet	1 tbsp	20	0.1	0.1	5.3	0.2
Pickle, cucumber, sour	1 large 4"	15	0.3	0.4	3.1	1.6
Pickle, cucumber, sweet	1 large 4"	158	0.3	0.5	42.9	1.5
Pickles, cucumber, dill	1 large 4"	24	0.2	0.8	5.5	1.6
Pie crust, graham-cracker, baked	1 pie crust	1037	52.3	8.8	136.9	3.2
Pie, apple	1 piece	411	19.4	3.7	57.5	0
Pie, blueberry	1 piece	290	12.5	2.2	43.6	1.3
Pie, cherry	1 piece	325	13.8	2.5	49.7	1
Pie, lemon meringue	1 piece	303	9.8	1.7	53.3	1.4
Pie, pecan	1 piece	452	20.9	4.5	64.6	4
Pie, pumpkin	1 piece	229	10.4	4.3	29.8	2.9
Pine nuts	1 oz. (167 kernels)	191	19.3	3.8	3.7	1

FOOD ITEM

FOOD ITEM	Serving Size	Cal.	Fat	Protein	Carbs	Fiber
P (cont.)						
Pineapple	1 fruit	227	0.6	2.5	59.6	6.6
Pineapple, canned	1 slice	15	0	0.2	3.9	0.4
Pita bread, whole wheat	1 pita	170	1.7	6.4	35.2	4.8
Pistachio nuts	1 oz (49 kernels)	161	13	6	7.6	2.9
Pizza, cheese	1 slice (3.7 oz.)	250	10	11	29	2
Pizza, pepperoni	1 slice (3.7 oz.)	288	15.2	11.7	26.1	1.7
Plantains	1 medium	218	0.7	2.3	57.1	4.1
Plums	1 fruit	30	0.2	0.5	7.5	0.9
Plums, canned	1 plum	19	0	0.2	5.1	0.4
Polenta	1/2 cup	220	2	2	24	1
Pomegranates	1 fruit	105	0.5	1.5	26.4	0.9
Popcorn cakes	1 cake	38	0.3	1	8	0.3
Popcorn, air-popped	1 cup	31	0.3	1	6.2	1.2
Popcorn, caramel-coated	1 oz	122	3.6	1.1	22.4	1.5
Popcorn, cheese	1 oz	58	3.7	1	5.7	1.1
Popcorn, oil-popped	1 cup	55	3.1	1	6.3	1.1
Popovers, dry mix	1 oz	105	1.2	2.9	20	0.5
Poppy seed	1 tsp	15	1.3	0.5	0.7	0.3
Pork, cured, breakfast strips, cooked	3 slices	156	12.4	9.8	0.3	0
Pork, cured, ham, extra lean, canned	3 oz	116	4.1	17.9	0.4	0
Pork, cured, ham, patties	1 patty	205	18.4	8.3	1.1	0
Pork, cured, ham, extra lean, cooked	3 oz	140	6.5	18.6	0.4	0
Pork, cured, salt pork, raw	1 oz	212	22.8	1.4	0	0
Pork, fresh ground, cooked	3 oz	252	17.6	21.8	0	0
Pork, leg, rump half, cooked	3 oz.	214	12.1	24.5	0	0
Pork, leg, shank half, cooked	3 oz	246	17	21.5	0	0
Pork, leg, whole, cooked	3 oz	232	14.9	22.8	0	0
Pork, loin, blade, cooked	3 oz	275	20.9	20.1	0	0
Pork, loin, center loin, cooked	3 oz	199	11.4	22.3	0	0
Pork, loin, center rib, cooked	3 oz	214	12.8	22.9	0	0
Pork, loin, sirloin, cooked	3 oz	176	8	24.2	0	0
Pork, loin, tenderloin, cooked	3 oz	147	5.1	23.6	0	0
Pork, loin, top loin, cooked	3 oz	192	9.7	24.4	0	0
Pork, loin, whole, cooked	3 oz	211	12.4	23	0	0
Pork, shoulder, arm, cooked	3 oz	238	18.1	17.3	0	0
Pork, shoulder, blade, cooked	3 oz	229	16	19.6	0	0
Pork, shoulder, whole, cooked	3 oz	248	18.2	19.8	0	0
Pork, spareribs, cooked	3 oz	337	25.7	24.7	0	0
Potato chips, barbecue	1 oz	139	9.2	2.2	14.9	1.2
Potato chips, cheese	1 oz	141	7.7	2.4	16.3	1.5
Potato chips, salted	1 oz	152	9.8	1.9	15	1.3
Potato chips, sour cream & onion	1 oz	151	9.6	2.3	14.6	1.5
Potato chips, reduced fat	1 oz	134	5.9	2	18.9	1.7
Potato chips, unsalted	1 oz	152	9.8	2	15	1.4
Potato flour	1 cup	571	0.5	11	132.9	9.4
Potato salad	1 cup	358	20.5	6.7	27.9	3.2
Potatoes	1 medium	164	0.2	4.3	37.2	4.7
Potatoes, baked, w/ skin	1 medium	160	0.2	4.3	36.5	3.8
Potatoes, baked, w/o skin	1 medium	143	0.2	2.8	33.3	3.3
Potatoes, mashed	1 cup	237	8.9	3.9	35.2	3.2

FOOD ITEM

	Serving Size	Cal.	Fat	Protein	Carbs	Fiber

P (cont.)

FOOD ITEM	Serving Size	Cal.	Fat	Protein	Carbs	Fiber
Potatoes, red	1 medium	153	0.3	4	33.9	3.6
Potatoes, russet	1 medium	168	0.2	4.6	38.5	2.8
Potatoes, scalloped	1 cup	211	9	7	26.4	4.7
Potatoes, white	1 medium	149	0.2	3.6	33.5	5.1
Pretzels, hard, plain, salted	1 oz.	108	0.9	2.6	22.4	0.9
Prune juice	8 fl oz.	180	0	2	43	3
Pudding, banana	1/2 cup	154	2.5	4	29	0
Pudding, chocolate	1/2 cup	154	2.8	4.6	27.7	0
Pudding, coconut cream	1/2 cup	157	3.3	4.2	28.2	0.1
Pudding, lemon	1/2 cup	157	2.5	4	29.7	0
Pudding, rice	1/2 cup	163	2.4	4.8	30.6	0.1
Pudding, tapioca	1/2 cup	154	2.4	4.2	28.7	0
Pudding, vanilla	1/2 cup	148	2.5	4.3	27.2	0
Pumpkin	1 cup	30	0.1	1.2	7.5	0.6
Pumpkin pie mix	1 cup	281	0.4	2.9	71.3	22.4
Pumpkin, canned	1 cup	83	0.7	2.7	19.8	7.1

R

FOOD ITEM	Serving Size	Cal.	Fat	Protein	Carbs	Fiber
Rabbit, cooked	3 oz	167	6.8	24.7	0	0
Radicchio	1 cup, shredded	9	0.1	0.6	1.8	0.4
Radishes	1 cup, sliced	19	0.1	0.8	3.9	1.9
Raisins	1 1/2 oz.	129	0.2	1.3	34	1.6
Raisins, golden	1 1/2 oz.	130	0.2	1.4	34.1	1.7
Raspberries	1 cup	64	0.8	1.5	14.7	8
Rhubarb	1 cup, diced	26	0.2	1.1	5.5	2.2
Rice cakes, brown rice, corn	1 cake	35	0.3	0.8	7.3	0.3
Rice cakes, brown rice, multi-grain	1 cake	35	0.3	0.8	7.2	0.3
Rice cakes, brown rice, plain	1 cake	35	0.3	0.7	7.3	0.4
Rice, brown, cooked	1 cup	218	1.6	4.5	45.8	3.5
Rice, white, cooked	1 cup	242	0.3	4.4	53.2	0.6
Rice, wild	1 cup	166	0.5	6.5	35	3
Rolls, dinner	1 roll	136	3.1	3.6	22.9	0.8
Rolls, dinner, wheat	1 roll	117	2.7	3.7	19.7	1.6
Rolls, dinner, whole-wheat	1 roll	114	2	3.7	21.9	3.2
Rolls, french	1 roll	119	1.8	3.7	21.5	0.1
Rolls, hamburger or hotdog	1 roll	120	1.9	4.1	21.3	0.9
Rolls, hard (incl. kaiser)	1 roll	126	1.8	4.2	22.6	1
Rolls, pumpernickel	1 roll	119	1.2	4.6	22.7	2.3
Rosemary	1 tsp	1	0	0	0.1	0.1
Rosemary, dried	1 tsp	4	0.2	0.1	0.8	0.5
Rum, 80 Proof	1 fl oz.	64	0	0	0	0
Rutabagas	1 cup, cubed	50	0.3	1.7	11.4	3.5
Rye	1 cup	566	4.2	24.9	117.9	24.7
Rye flour, dark	1 cup	415	3.4	18	88	28.9
Rye flour, light	1 cup	374	1.4	8.6	81.8	14.9
Rye flour, medium	1 cup	361	1.8	9.6	79	14.9

S

FOOD ITEM	Serving Size	Cal.	Fat	Protein	Carbs	Fiber
Sage, ground	1 tsp	2	0.1	0.1	0.4	0.3
Sake	1 fl oz	39	0	0.1	1.5	0

FOOD ITEM

FOOD ITEM	Serving Size	Cal.	Fat	Protein	Carbs	Fiber
Salad dressing, 1000 island	1 tbsp	58	5.5	0.2	2.3	0.1
Salad dressing, bacon & tomato	1 tbsp	49	5.3	0.3	0.3	0
Salad dressing, blue cheese	1 tbsp	77	8	0.7	1.1	0
Salad dressing, caesar	1 tbsp	78	8.5	0.2	0.5	0
Salad dressing, coleslaw	1 tbsp	61	5.2	0.1	3.7	0
Salad dressing, french	1 tbsp	71	7	0.1	2.4	0
Salad dressing, honey dijon	1 tbsp	57.5	5	0.5	3	0.5
Salad dressing, italian	1 tbsp	43	4.2	0.1	1.5	0
Salad dressing, mayo-based	1 tbsp	57	4.9	0.1	3.5	0
Salad dressing, mayonnaise	1 tbsp	103	11.7	0	0	0
Salad dressing, peppercorn	1 tbsp	76	8.2	0.2	0.5	0
Salad dressing, ranch	1 tbsp	25	0	0	0	0
Salad dressing, russian	1 tbsp	76	7.8	0.2	1.6	0
Salad, chicken	6 oz.	420	33	45	11	1.5
Salad, egg	6 oz.	300	23	20	14	0.5
Salad, prima pasta	6 oz.	360	30	4.8	18	2.5
Salad, seafood w/ crab & shrimp	6 oz.	420	34	0	20	0
Salad, tuna	6 oz.	450	36	16	14	0
Salami, cooked, turkey	1 oz	37.7	2.3	0.7	0	0
Salami, dry, pork or beef	3 slices	104	8.1	6.3	1	0
Salami, italian pork	1 oz	119	10.4	6.1	0.3	0
Salsa, w/ oil	2 tbsp	40	3	0	8	0
Salsa, w/o oil	2 tbsp	15	0	0	3.5	0
Salt	1 tbsp	0	0	0	0	0
Sauce, alfredo	1/4 cup	120	11	15	3	2
Sauce, bbq	1 cup	188	4.5	4.5	32	3
Sauce, cheese	1 cup	479	36.3	25.1	13.3	0.2
Sauce, cranberry	1 cup	418	0.4	0.6	107.8	2.8
Sauce, hollandaise	1 cup	62	1.5	2.3	10.3	0.2
Sauce, honey mustard	1 tbsp	30	1	0	5	0
Sauce, marinara	1 cup	185	6	4.9	28.2	1
Sauce, salsa	1 cup	70	0.4	4	16.2	4.1
Sauce, soy	1 tbsp	10	0	0	0	0
Sauce, steak	1 tbsp	25	0	0	6	0
Sauce, teriyaki	1 tbsp	15	0	17	0	0
Sauce, tomato chili	1 cup	284	0.8	6.8	54	16.1
Sauce, worcestershire	1 cup	184	0	0	53.5	0
Sauerkraut	1/2 cup	25	0	1	5	4
Sausage, italian pork, raw	1 link	391	35.4	16.1	0.7	0
Sausage, pork	1 link	85	7.4	4.2	0	0
Sausage, smoked linked, pork	1 link	265	21.6	15.1	1.4	0
Sausage, turkey	1 link	0	0	0	0	0
Savory, ground	1 tsp	4	0.1	0.1	1	0.6
Scallops	1 scallop	26	0.2	5	0.7	0
Seaweed, dried	1 oz.	50	0	0	13	0
Sesame seeds, dried	1 tbsp	52	4.5	1.6	2.1	1.1
Shallots	1 tbsp, chopped	7	0	0.3	1.7	0
Shortening	1 tbsp	113	12.8	0	0	0
Shrimp, mixed species, raw	1 medium piece	6	0.1	1.2	0.1	0
Snacks, cheese puffs or twists	1 oz.	157	9.7	2.1	15.2	0.3

FOOD ITEM

S (cont.)

FOOD ITEM	Serving Size	Cal.	Fat	Protein	Carbs	Fiber
Soda, club	12 fl oz.	0	0	0	0	0
Soda, cream	12 fl oz.	252	0	0	65.7	0
Soda, diet cola	12 fl oz.	0	0	0	0	0
Soda, ginger-ale	12 fl oz.	166	0	0	42.8	0
Soda, lemon-lime	12 fl oz.	196	0	0	51.1	0
Soda, regular, w/ caffeine	12 fl oz.	155	0	0.2	39.8	0
Soda, regular, w/o caffeine	12 fl oz.	207	0	0.2	52.9	0
Soda, root beer	12 fl oz.	202	0	0	52.3	0
Soda, tonic water	12 fl oz.	166	0	0	42.9	0
Soup, beef broth	1 cup	29	0	5.3	1.7	0
Soup, beef stroganoff	1 cup	235	11	12.2	21.6	1.4
Soup, beef vegetable	1 cup	82	1.9	2.9	13.1	0.5
Soup, chicken broth	1 cup	39	1.3	4.9	0.9	0
Soup, chicken noodle	1 cup	75	2.4	4	9.3	0.7
Soup, chicken vegetable	1 cup	75	2.8	3.6	8.5	1
Soup, chicken w/ dumplings	1 cup	96	5.5	5.6	6	0.5
Soup, clam chowder	1 cup	95	2.8	4.8	12.4	1.5
Soup, cream of chicken	1 cup	117	7.3	3.4	9.2	0.2
Soup, cream of mushroom	1 cup	129	8.9	2.3	9.3	0.5
Soup, cream of potato	1 cup	149	6.4	5.7	17	0.5
Soup, minestrone	1 cup	82	2.5	4.2	11.2	1
Soup, split-pea w/ham	1 cup	190	4.4	10.3	27.9	2.3
Soup, tomato	1 cup	161	6	6.1	22.3	2.7
Soup, vegetarian	1 cup	72	1.9	2.1	11.9	0.5
Sour cream	1 tbsp	26	2.5	0.4	0.5	0
Sour cream, fat free	1 tbsp	9	0	0.3	1.8	0
Sour cream, reduced fat	1 tbsp	22	1.7	0.8	0.8	0
Soy milk	1 cup	127	4.7	10.9	12	3.2
Soy protein isolate	1 oz	96	1	22.9	2.1	1.6
Soybeans, green, cooked	1 cup	254	11.5	22.2	19.8	7.6
Soybeans, nuts, roasted	1/4 cup	194	9.2	17	14	3.4
Soyburger	1 patty	125	4.1	12.5	9.3	3.2
Spaghetti, cooked	1 cup	197	0.9	6.6	39.6	2.4
Spaghetti, spinach, cooked	1 cup	182	0.8	6.4	36.6	2.4
Spaghetti, whole-wheat, cooked	1 cup	174	0.7	7.4	37.1	6.3
Spinach	1 cup	7	0.1	0.9	1.1	0.7
Squab, boneless, raw	1 squab	585	47.4	36.8	0	0
Squab, skinless, raw	1 squab	239	12.6	29.4	0	0
Squash, summer	1 cup, sliced	18	0.2	1.4	3.8	1.2
Squash, winter	1 cup, cubed	39	0.2	1.1	10	1.7
Squid, mixed species, raw	1 oz	26	0.4	4.4	0.9	0
Stock, beef	1 cup	31	0.2	4.7	2.9	0
Stock, chicken	1 cup	86	2.9	6	8.5	0
Stock, fish	1 cup	40	1.9	5.3	0	0
Strawberries	1 cup	49	0.5	1	11.7	3
Succotash	1 piece	0	0	0	0	0
Sugar, brown	1 tsp	12	0	0	3.1	0
Sugar, granulated	1 tsp	16	0	0	4.2	0
Sugar, maple	1 tsp	11	0	0	2.7	0
Sugar, powdered	1 tsp	10	0	0	2.5	0

FOOD ITEM

FOOD ITEM	Serving Size	Cal.	Fat	Protein	Carbs	Fiber
S (cont.)						
Sunflower seeds	1 tbsp	45	10	4	1.5	5
Sweet potato	1 cup, cubed	114	0.1	2.1	26.8	4
Syrup, chocolate	1 tbsp	66.5	1.7	0.8	11.9	0.5
Syrup, dark corn	1 tbsp	57	0	0	15.5	0
Syrup, grenadine	1 tbsp	53	0	0	13.3	0
Syrup, light corn	1 tbsp	59	0	0	15.9	0
Syrup, maple	1 tbsp	52	0	0	13.4	0
Syrup, pancake	1 tbsp	47	0	0	12.3	0.1
T						
Taco shell, hard	1 shell	55	3	2	6	0
Tangerines	1 large	52	0.3	0.8	13.1	1.8
Tarragon, dried	1 tsp	2	0	0.1	0.3	0
Tea, instant	1 cup	2	0	0.1	0.4	0
Thyme	1 tsp	1	0	0	0.2	0.1
Thyme, dried	1 tsp	3	0.1	0.1	0.6	0.4
Tofu, firm	1/2 cup	183	11	19.9	5.4	2.9
Tofu, fried	1 piece	35	2.6	2.2	1.4	0.5
Tofu, soft	1/2 cup	75.5	4.6	8.1	2.2	0.2
Tomato juice, canned, with salt	6 fl oz	31	0.1	1.4	7.7	0.7
Tomato juice, canned, without salt	6 fl oz	30	0.1	1.2	7.8	0.7
Tomato paste, canned	1/2 cup	107	0.6	5.7	24.8	5.9
Tomato sauce, canned	1 cup	78	0.6	3.2	18.1	3.7
Tomatoes, canned, crushed	1 cup	82	0.7	4.2	18.6	4.8
Tomatoes, green	1 cup, chopped	41	0.4	2.2	9.2	2
Tomatoes, orange	1 cup, chopped	25	0.3	1.8	5	1.4
Tomatoes, red	1 cup, chopped	32	0.4	1.6	7.1	2.2
Tomatoes, sun-dried	1 cup, chopped	139	1.6	7.6	30.1	6.6
Toppings, butterscotch or caramel	2 tbsp	103	0	0.6	27	0.4
Toppings, marshmallow crème	2 tbsp	132	0.1	0.3	32.3	0
Toppings, nuts in syrup	2 tbsp	184	9	1.8	23.8	0.9
Toppings, pineapple	2 tbsp	106	0	0	27.9	0.2
Toppings, strawberry	2 tbsp	107	0	0.1	27.8	0.3
Tortilla chips, plain	1 oz.	142	7.4	1.9	17.8	1.8
Tortilla, corn	1 tortilla	45	0.5	2	9	3
Tortilla, flour	1 tortilla	160	3	18	28	3
Trail mix	1/4 cup	173.2	11	5	16.8	3
Turkey, deli sliced, white meat	1 oz.	30	1	5	0.5	0
Turkey, back, skinless, boneless, raw	1/2 back	180	5.3	31	0	0
Turkey, breast, boneless, raw	1/2 breast	541	11.5	102.9	0	0
Turkey, breast, skinless, boneless, raw	1/2 breast	433	2.5	95.9	0	0
Turkey, dark meat, boneless, raw	1/2 turkey	686	25.5	106.7	0	0
Turkey, dark meat, skinless, boneless, raw	1/2 turkey	532	12.8	98	0	0
Turkey, leg, boneless, raw	1 leg	412	12.5	70.3	0	0
Turkey, leg, skinless, boneless, raw	1 leg	355	7.8	67	0	0
Turkey, wing, boneless, raw	1 wing	204	9.9	26.7	0	0
Turkey, wing, skinless, boneless, raw	1 wing	95	1	20.2	0	0
Turkey, young hen, back, boneless, raw	1/2 back	650	47.5	52.2	0	0
Turkey, young hen, breast, boneless, raw	1/2 breast	1460	72.5	189	0	0
Turkey, young hen, dark meat, boneless, raw	1/2 turkey	1056	39.6	163	0	0

FOOD ITEM

FOOD ITEM	Serving Size	Cal.	Fat	Protein	Carbs	Fiber
T (cont.)						
Turkey, young hen, leg, boneless, raw	1 leg	991	49.2	127.7	0	0
Turkey, young hen, wing, boneless, raw	1 wing	470	31.1	44.6	0	0
Turkey, young tom, back, boneless, raw	1/2 back	938	58.4	96.8	0	0
Turkey, young tom, breast, boneless, raw	1/2 breast	2701	113.4	392.9	0	0
Turkey, young tom, dark meat, boneless, raw	1/2 turkey	1884	63	307	0	0
Turkey, young tom, leg, boneless, raw	1 leg	1740	78.2	241.1	0	0
Turkey, young tom, wing, boneless, raw	1 wing	654	39	71.2	0	0
Turnip greens	1 cup, chopped	18	0.2	0.8	3.9	1.8
Turnips	1 cup, cubed	36	0.1	1.2	8.4	2.3
V						
Vanilla extract	1 tbsp	37	0	0	1.6	0
Veal, breast, raw	1 oz	59	4.2	5	0	0
Veal, cubed, raw	1 oz	31	0.7	5.7	0	0
Veal, ground, raw	1 oz	41	1.9	5.5	0	0
Veal, leg, raw	1 oz	33	0.9	5.9	0	0
Veal, loin, raw	1 oz	46	2.6	5.4	0	0
Veal, rib, raw	1 oz	46	2.6	5.3	0	0
Veal, shank, raw	1 oz	32	1	5.4	0	0
Veal, shoulder, arm, raw	1 oz	37	1.5	5.5	0	0
Veal, shoulder, blade, raw	1 oz	37	1.5	5.5	0	0
Veal, shoulder, whole, raw	1 oz	37	1.5	5.5	0	0
Veal, sirloin, raw	1 oz	43	2.2	5.4	0	0
Vegetable juice	8 fl oz	50	0	2	12	2
Vinegar	1 tbsp	2	0	0	0.8	0
W						
Waffles, plain	1 waffle	218	10.6	5.9	24.7	0
Walnuts	1 oz. (14 halves)	185	18.5	4.3	3.9	1.9
Wasabi root	1 cup, sliced	142	0.8	6.2	30.6	10.1
Water chestnuts, chinese	1/2 cup, sliced	60	0.1	0.9	14.8	1.9
Watercress	1 cup, chopped	4	0	0.8	0.4	0.2
Watermelon	1 cup, diced	46	0.2	0.9	11.5	0.6
Wheat bran	1 cup	125	2.5	9	37.4	24.8
Wheat flour, whole grain	1 cup	407	2.2	16.4	87.1	14.6
Wheat germ	1 cup	414	11.2	26.6	59.6	15.2
Whipped cream	1 cup	154	13.3	1.9	7.5	0
Wine, cooking	1 tsp	2	0	0	0.3	0
Wine, red	3-1/2 oz. glass	74	0	0.2	1.8	0
Wine, rose	3-1/2 oz. glass	73	0	0.2	1.4	0
Wine, white	3-1/2 oz. glass	70	0	0.1	0.8	0
Yam	1 cup, cubed	177	0.3	2.3	41.8	6.1
Yeast, active, dry	1 tsp	12	0.2	1.5	1.5	0.8
Yogurt, fruit, low-fat	8 oz. container	118	0.3	5.5	23.8	0
Yogurt, fruit, whole milk	8 oz. container	250	6	9	38	0
Yogurt, plain, low-fat	8 oz. container	110	4	7.9	7	0
Yogurt, plain, whole milk	8 oz. container	138	7.4	12	10.6	0
Z						
Zucchini	1 medium	45	0	2	10	1